Dementia Myth
Most Patients with Dementia Are Curable

Dr Vernon Coleman MB ChB DSc FRSA

Published by EMJ Books

Dedication
To Antoinette who cares
With all my love as always.

The author
Vernon Coleman MB ChB DSc FRSA has been a successful campaigning medical writer for 50 years. He has written over 100 books which have sold over two million copies in the UK alone, and been translated into 25 languages. For more information please see www.vernoncoleman.com or visit Vernon Coleman's author page on Amazon.

Contents

Preface
Part One: The Process
Chapter One: An Introduction to the Dementia Myth
Chapter Two: How Critical Doctors Are Silenced
Chapter Three: The Power of Modern Charities
Chapter Four: The NHS Misleads
Chapter Five: Medical Journals – Corrupt and Misleading
Part Two: The Causes of dementia
Chapter One: Prescription drugs
Chapter Two: Inadequate vitamin B12
Chapter Three: Normal Pressure Hydrocephalus
Chapter Four: Alzheimer's disease
Appendices
Appendix One: Case history: Antoinette Coleman
Appendix Two: Facts about vitamin B12 deficiency
Appendix Three: Symptoms and diseases caused by low Vitamin B12
Appendix Four: Case histories: patients with normal pressure hydrocephalus
Appendix Five: Homocysteine and Alzheimer's disease
Appendix Six: High blood pressure and Alzheimer's disease
Appendix Seven: Paracetamol and Alzheimer's disease
Appendix Eight: Alzheimer's disease financial incentive
Appendix Nine: Alzheimer's and death
Appendix Ten: When demented patients wander
Appendix Eleven: Recommendations

Preface

The diagnosis, treatment and reporting of dementia is a massive and previously unrecognised scandal. The staggering fact is that most cases of dementia could probably be cured in a week or two – maybe a little longer with some patients. Anyone who says otherwise is either woefully misinformed or a drug company mouthpiece.

Around the world there are estimated to be around 50 million people suffering from dementia – though this figure is probably on the low side. One half of all the patients admitted to nursing homes are said to be suffering from dementia of one sort or another.

Millions of patients who have been diagnosed with dementia are being looked after by their families. Many family members have had to abandon their jobs and their normal lives in order to find the necessary time to provide care for their loved ones. Millions more patients have been dumped in hospitals and nursing homes where they sit or lie, waiting to die.

No one knows how many millions of as yet undiagnosed individuals are struggling to cope with dementia, either alone or with the help of relatives, friends and neighbours.

The commonest diagnosis for all these patients is Alzheimer's disease. It is widely reputed that two thirds of patients with dementia are suffering from Alzheimer's. Indeed, Alzheimer's has in many countries become the default diagnosis. If a patient has dementia then they will be assumed to be suffering from Alzheimer's and little or no effort will be made to find any other diagnosis. The drug companies, the big charities, the media and even some doctors seem to promote the view that the words 'dementia' and 'Alzheimer's' are pretty well interchangeable.

The prognosis for those diagnosed as suffering from Alzheimer's disease is a gloomy one for, despite many promises, there is still no cure for this disease, nor is there any sign of a cure on the horizon. Drug companies have produced a number of prescription only drugs recommended for use with Alzheimer patients, and alternative health care practitioners produce new remedies on an almost daily basis.

Despite all the promotion given to Alzheimer's disease, there is however, clear evidence that many so-called dementia sufferers who have been diagnosed as suffering from Alzheimer's disease have been misdiagnosed. They are suffering from something quite different and could be cured – often completely and frequently within weeks or even days.

This short book is intended simply to draw attention to this scandal and to provide pointers for those who feel that a loved one may have been misdiagnosed. My aim is not to provide a comprehensive guide to any of the diseases which cause dementia but, rather, to offer direction for those who might otherwise be led into a fateful diagnosis when other more hopeful possibilities might exist.

Some patients who have dementia will, of course, have Alzheimer's disease, and will be incurable. But if just one patient can be rescued from a faulty diagnosis and returned to an active, productive life then writing this book will have been well worthwhile.

Dr Vernon Coleman MB ChB DSc FRSA

Part One: The Process

Chapter One

An Introduction to the Dementia Myth

Some people believe that dementia is a normal part of the ageing process (hence the term 'senile dementia'), but it is not. That is one of the many myths about dementia.

There are hundreds of thousands of people in their 80s and 90s who still have all their mental faculties intact; thousands have gone on to achieve great things in their advanced years. Dementia is neither a natural nor an inevitable consequence of ageing. (I wrote a short book called *Climbing Trees at 112* which list the achievements of a variety of elder citizens.)

The second myth is that dementia is not itself a disease. The word 'dementia' is a general word for the symptoms displayed as a result of a number of different diseases. (In much the same way that 'cancer' and 'infection' aren't specific diseases.)

When someone displays symptoms of dementia, it's the doctor's job to identify the underlying cause.

Besides Alzheimer's, other disorders that can cause dementia include: advanced syphilis, vitamin B12 deficiency, Huntington's disease, Down's Syndrome, Pick's disease, strokes, Lewy Body disease, late-multiple sclerosis, brain tumours, hormone deficiencies, chronic alcoholism, drug abuse (of both illegal and prescription drugs), head injuries, and idiopathic normal pressure hydrocephalus.

Nearly half of all individuals with Parkinson's disease develop dementia, though this usually occurs about 10 or 15 years after the disease has first been diagnosed. Dementia can also occur in a condition called Creutzfeldt-Jakob disease and Variant Creutzfeldt-Jakob disease. Dementia also sometimes occurs in the late stages of human immunodeficiency virus (HIV). And there is dementia pugilistica, also known as chronic progressive traumatic encephalopathy. This is a disorder which develops in people who have repeated head injuries – boxers and American football players, for example – and which produces symptoms similar to Parkinson's disease. The boxer Muhammad Ali may, in my opinion, have been suffering from this disorder for the last years of his life. These individuals may also develop normal pressure hydrocephalus. And there is a condition known as vascular dementia.

Quite a number of the less common types of dementia are treatable. So, for example, patients who have developed dementia as a result of having a treatable brain tumour, patients who are suffering from poisoning (as a result of toxins such as lead or mercury), patients who have syphilis, Lyme disease and other infective disorders and patents who have myxoedema (an underactive thyroid gland) may all recover when their conditions are treated. Patients who develop dementia after a sudden head injury may also make a good recovery.

Some of these are disorders about which many doctors, including specialists know next to nothing. Relatives and friends of patients with dementia need to push hard to make sure that alternative causes of dementia are not ignored or forgotten for it is crucial to remember that some of these disorders are treatable and a diagnosis of Alzheimer's should never be made until all other disorders have been excluded.

To find the underlying cause of a p a t i e n t ' s symptoms, a doctor needs to do quite a battery of tests. She or he may refer the patient to a neurologist at a hospital or he or she may make a diagnosis based on symptoms and medical history alone. Whatever happens, the diagnosis should not be made without certain basic investigations being conducted, and treatable conditions must be excluded before a diagnosis of (for example) Alzheimer's disease is made. It is sloppy and unprofessional to make a diagnosis of Alzheimer's as a default diagnosis.

To claim that dementia is incurable is as absurd as saying that all people with broken legs will never walk again or that all patients with chest infections will die. It is cruel, manipulative scaremongering, and those who repeat this nonsense should be ashamed of themselves and their ignorance.

As I pointed out above (but make no apology for repeating), the truth is that 'dementia' is a word like 'cancer' and 'infection'.

There are many causes of cancer.

There are many causes of infection.

And there are many causes of dementia. And some of those causes are curable or, at the very least, controllable if they are properly diagnosed and well-treated.

Parkinson's disease can cause dementia but drugs may help. Huntington's disease can cause dementia and although it is not curable, there are medicines available which may help reduce the severity of symptoms. Alcoholism can cause dementia but, as millions can confirm, alcoholism is a controllable disease. Then there is dementia caused by vascular disease. This is estimated to affect around 150,000 people in the UK alone and although there is no cure, there are drugs available which can slow down the progress of the disease. Many patients who are depressed show signs of dementia which will disappear when their depression lifts. Patients who have normal pressure hydrocephalus show clear signs of dementia but they can be permanently cured with a simple operation. Hundreds of thousands of patients appear demented because they have been over-dosed with tranquillisers and sedatives. These patients will recover completely if their unnecessary medication is stopped or reduced. And hundreds of thousands of patients who have all the symptoms of dementia, and who may have been given the default diagnosis of Alzheimer's disease, will show a dramatic improvement in a couple of weeks if all they have wrong with them is an undiagnosed vitamin B12 deficiency – treatable with simple injections of the missing vitamin.

And there are many other causes of dementia.

The point is that dementia is not the same thing as Alzheimer's disease and anyone who suggests otherwise is grossly irresponsible – whether they are a doctor, a nurse, a charity worker or a drug company employee.

The dementia/Alzheimer's disease scandal is one of the biggest medical scandals in history and I suspect that current policies are laying doctors, hospitals and laboratories wide open to the largest class action lawsuit in medical history.

Though ignorance and laziness on the part of doctors, and as a result of deliberate misinformation spread by a deadly combination of drug companies and specialist charities, hundreds of thousands of patients have been given a default diagnosis of Alzheimer's disease without proper investigations ever being conducted.

The hidden, underlying problem is that medical policy relating to the classification, diagnosis and treatment of dementia is defined and directed by drug companies which have for some years controlled the medical establishment and which run medicine so that their own commercial interests are best served. And that means encouraging doctors to make diagnoses which are commercially advantageous and then promoting and selling large quantities of drugs which are expensive and profitable but often largely useless. (Making a profit is, of course, the raison d'etre of the drug industry. The medical establishment, which has sold out to the drug industry, is far more culpable.)

I will return to the question of dementia in a moment but I need a short diversion here to point out that it is not, of course, merely in the diagnosis and treatment of dementia that drug companies have established advantageous principles.

The massive increase in the number of children diagnosed as suffering from asthma is a direct result of drug company propaganda. Most of the children so diagnosed have merely suffered an isolated incidence of wheezing. But, once diagnosed as asthmatic they will be given regular supplies of tablets and inhalers and they will become life-long profit bases for the industry.

Most patients who have high blood pressure would find that their blood pressure levels returned to normal if they lost excess weight and learned to deal more effectively with the stress in their lives. But in order for the drug companies to make profits, general practitioners must prescribe daily drugs. And so that is the default form of treatment.

Patients who are overweight are given pills rather than dietary advice. Patients who are anxious or suffering from stress are given endless repeat prescriptions for tranquillisers or anti-depressants despite the availability of evidence showing that these drugs are dangerously addictive. Patients who suffer from mild pain are given repeat prescriptions for addictive opiate drugs. And so it goes.

My first book, published in 1975, was called *The Medicine Men* and in it I explained how the drug companies control the medical profession. Since then the situation has changed only in that the hold the drug industry has over the medical establishment has tightened.

The majority of senior doctors working in medicine have received substantial amounts of drug company money – either in cash or gifts, and a couple of decades ago I exposed the astonishing fact that at that time just about every doctor appointed to supervise the profession's use of drugs, and its relationship with the drug industry, had received money or gifts from drug companies. I doubt if things are any different today.

Medical journals exist only because of the huge amounts of money they receive from drug companies in the form of advertising. Medical lectures and symposia are organised with the financial help of drug companies. Most postgraduate education is influenced, controlled or organised by the pharmaceutical industry.

That's the end of the diversion into the background explanation of the extent of the influence of the pharmaceutical industry.

Now, I'll go back to dementia.

The result of the fact that the drug industry controls the medical profession is that the diagnosis and treatment of patients with dementia is completely controlled by a ruthless industry which, via clever marketing campaigns and the crafty use of charities, has quite different aims to those of patients.

And so, around the world, we have the tragic situation in which millions of patients who currently have symptoms of dementia, who have been dismissively labelled with the default diagnosis of Alzheimer's disease, and who are living out their days in institutions where they have no freedom and no responsibility for their own lives, could have been cured and could be enjoying the final years and decades of their lives.

The drug companies get away with this for two primary and simple reasons.

First, medical school departments are largely run by specialists in obscure and often untreatable diseases who often ignore disorders such as vitamin B12 deficiency and normal pressure hydrocephalus because these are relatively common and straightforward to treat disorders. Doctors who specialise in these conditions are likely to find that they don't merit drug company sponsored invitations to foreign conferences in fascinating places. These are not disorders which merit massive drug company investment. Drug companies have a particular affection for common, chronic and incurable diseases such as arthritis, diabetes and high blood pressure because they are exceptionally profitable. And so, for example, drug companies make far more money if young patients who are suffering from vitamin B12 deficiency are diagnosed as suffering from multiple sclerosis. (Multiple sclerosis and vitamin B12 deficiency produce almost identical symptoms.) Drug therapy for multiple sclerosis is enormously expensive (and profitable) whereas the profits involved in the treatment of vitamin B12 deficiency are measured in pennies.

Second, the post graduate medical education of general practitioners is effectively controlled by the pharmaceutical industry which sponsors lectures and buys absurdly over-priced advertising in medical journals.

As far as dementia is concerned, the result is that millions of patients who are now spending the remaining years requiring constant nursing care could and should be living independent, full lives.

Millions of people who are bedridden in hospital, or living vegetative, sedated lives in nursing homes could be working or enjoying the retirement years to which they no doubt looked forward.

And millions of relatives who have chosen to abandon their own lives in order to provide adequate, loving care for their relations should now be continuing with their own lives.

The cost to individuals, and to the community at large, is too large to measure. The emotional cost is phenomenal. And the blunt financial cost is horrifying and has to be measured in tens of billions. There is the cost of providing home or institutional care for patients requiring constant attention and there is the cost of purchasing the largely useless pharmaceuticals sold by the greediest and most ruthless industry man has ever created. (I have previously pointed out that the international pharmaceutical industry makes the Columbian drug barons look positively caring and philanthropic.)

All this happens because venal and easily influenced medical practitioners have betrayed their profession and misdiagnosed millions of patients. And they have misdiagnosed those patients because they have been misled (brain washed would, perhaps, be a better word) by the international pharmaceutical industry.

Is that not a scandal of brobdingnagian proportions?

Medicine today doesn't need more innovation, more research, more technology or more digitalisation. It needs, desperately needs, more integrity and more honesty.

And until the medical profession breaks free of drug company control, and acquires a little integrity and honesty, then patients are on their own and must take control of their own lives and their own illnesses.

Today, the result of the propaganda efforts of the pharmaceutical industry (and the charities with which the industry is now linked) is that there is no doubt that if you asked 1,000 people to name the commonest cause of dementia at least 999 of them would say 'Alzheimer's disease'. Indeed, most of the 1,000 would probably tell you that 'dementia' is just another word for 'Alzheimer's' and that the two are synonymous.

Alarmingly, a similar result would be obtained if you asked 1,000 doctors to name the commonest cause of dementia.

And, of course, much the same result would be obtained if you asked the same question of 1,000 specialist medical journalists working for print and broadcast media.

They would, of course, all be completely wrong.

Despite the widespread consequences of the propaganda machine, Alzheimer's disease is not the same thing as dementia.

And, despite everything we have been led to believe, Alzheimer's disease isn't even the commonest cause of dementia. (I confess that I used to believe this assertion. But it simply isn't true. It is a convenient piece of marketing propaganda. Many of those doomed with a diagnosis of Alzheimer's disease have something else wrong with them. And the 'something else' is usually curable.)

As I have pointed out, these myths about dementia and Alzheimer's disease have not come into being by accident. On the contrary, they are the result of a very deliberate campaign of propaganda and misinformation. And the propaganda has been managed very deliberately and ruthlessly and with absolute no regard for the health of patients. I make no apology for repeating this assertion. The fact is that the myths about dementia are frighteningly deep rooted and devastatingly shocking and the rebuttal of the lies cannot be over-emphasised.

The cheats and fraudsters in the drug companies and the big charities have doubtless been helped by the fact that there is no test for Alzheimer's disease. The drug companies love diseases, especially chronic diseases, which cannot be proven because there is no specific, reliable diagnostic test.

This absence of a simple and incontrovertible test is very convenient for the drug companies and for the large charities which tend to work alongside them. The absence of a single, reliable test has made it damnably easy for the drug companies and the charities to ensure that Alzheimer's is the default diagnosis made by doctors.

(The Alzheimer charities have been invaluable for the drug companies, for their apparent independence has made it easy for them to convince the media around the world to accept the myth that 'dementia' and 'Alzheimer's' are interchangeable. The Alzheimer charities are often closely linked to drug companies which make expensive and profitable 'remedies' for use in the control of patients with Alzheimer's. Naturally, the charities are pumped full of cash by the grateful drug companies. I explain later on in this book precisely how the drug companies manage to buy and control so many charities. This sort of activity is not, of course, confined to charities dealing with dementia and Alzheimer's disease.)

For purely commercial reasons, the drug companies (and their chums the big Alzheimer charities) are desperately keen to convince people that Alzheimer's and dementia are the same thing. It is in the interest of the drug companies to diagnose every case of dementia as Alzheimer's disease. We can't blame the drug companies. We have to remember that their only reason for existence is to make money. They don't exist to help patients get better. They don't exist to make the world a better place. They are profit-making machines.

The blunt bottom line fact is that drug companies don't want patients to be diagnosed with disorders such as vitamin B12 deficiency or with normal pressure hydrocephalus because they won't make money out of those patients.

It is, of course, all about the money.

There are a number of drugs on the market for the 'treatment' of Alzheimer's disease. The drugs available are expensive and in my view they do little or no good; they certainly don't 'cure' patients. But obviously, drug company profits will rise as the number of patients being treated rises.

Doctors are easy to bribe for several reasons.

First, I am afraid that most modern doctors have little sense of vocation. You can see this in the way that GPs in the UK leapt at the chance to avoid providing their patients with night time and weekend cover. If doctors really cared for their patients they would have happily continued with the established system which ensured that patient care was provided around the clock. Today, medicine is a business and most doctors are in it for what they can get out of it rather than what they can put into it. (This means, inevitably, that patients must take control of their own lives and take a real interest in their own healthcare. It is no longer safe for a patient to be a passive patient; allowing themselves to be treated, as required, and to be swept along by the system.)

Second, doctors who dare to question the way the system works are likely to be crushed. So, for example, doctors who question the power of the pharmaceutical industry, or any aspect of the provision of medical services, are quickly destroyed so that the system (profitable for drug companies and doctors) can continue unchanged. I find it difficult to think of a profession which suppresses original thought more efficiently or more ruthlessly than the medical profession. I have shown elsewhere in this book precisely how doctors can be crushed if they try to rock the boat.

Third, and probably most important of all, medicine is designed and practised to treat sick patients. It isn't designed to keep patients healthy and to prevent illness. And it isn't designed to get them well again. It is designed to provide treatment. If the modern medical system were an individual human being, it would be disappointed if a patient got better because a patient who gets better no longer needs treatment. The system exists, is fed and grows by the extent of the people needing treatment. This may sound pedantic but it isn't. And it is a result of the fact that the medical profession is controlled by the pharmaceutical industry. Remember: the pharmaceutical industry doesn't ever want people to get better. If the pharmaceutical industry found a secret pill that would cure everyone in a day then it would destroy the recipe for that pill. The pharmaceutical industry would be ruined if someone found a cure for cancer, a cure for heart disease or a reliable cure for infection.

Moreover, in the UK the Government helps the drug companies in their crooked aim by bribing doctors to diagnose Alzheimer's every time they see a patient who is confused, bewildered or showing signs of dementia.

And every time a doctor stamps a diagnosis of Alzheimer's on a patient's records, she or he increases the official incidence of Alzheimer's and helps to turn the myth into reality.

GPs in the UK are willing participants in this fraud because (for reasons which are quite incomprehensible) the Government gives them money every time they diagnose Alzheimer's disease. GPs receive no bonus if they diagnose vitamin B12 deficiency or normal pressure hydrocephalus. They receive no bonus for finding a treatable form of dementia but they are rewarded by the taxpayers for diagnosing a form of dementia which will involve huge costs for taxpayers and huge profits for drug companies.

It is important to remember that the drug companies favour Alzheimer's disease for very simple reasons.

First, Alzheimer's disease tends to be chronic. It lasts for years. It does not usually kill patients. (Most patients who are said to have died of Alzheimer's disease have died of something else – usually an untreated chest infection.) The drug companies love chronic diseases. Providing pills for patients who need medication for years is far more profitable than providing pills for a one or two week course. This is why drug companies are far more enthusiastic about finding new treatments for arthritis or high blood pressure, both usually regarded as long-term disorders, than they are about finding new treatments for infections. A new antibiotic is likely to be prescribed for a week or two weeks. A new painkiller, promoted as suitable for treating patients with arthritis (whether or not there is any evidence for the claim) is likely to prove enormously profitable. Drugs which are marketed in competition with existing products are known in the business as 'me-too' drugs.

Second, most of the other major causes of dementia do not need expensive drugs. Patients who have acquired the symptoms of dementia because they are short of vitamin B12 can be treated with very inexpensive injections of B12.

Patients who appear demented because they are being heavily dosed with tranquillisers or sleeping tablets will recover if their drugs are reduced or stopped. (This is particularly unpopular with drug companies because it doesn't just prevent future drug sales but actually reduces drug sales and therefore has a devastating effect on profitability.) And patients who have normal pressure hydrocephalus can be cured with a very simple and cheap operation which requires virtually no input from the pharmaceutical industry – leaving absolutely no chance of profits for drug companies.

The result of all this is that the people who are profiting from the growth in the incidence of Alzheimer's (this includes drug companies and those charities which have close links with drug companies) want you to believe that when a patient shows symptoms and signs of dementia, the default diagnosis must be Alzheimer's disease. Indeed, they would rather no other options were even considered.

If everyone who is demented is assumed to be suffering from Alzheimer's disease then the profits for drug companies flogging medicines for the 'treatment' of Alzheimer's patients will soar. Drug companies (and the charities which work with them) have a vested interest in suppressing the diagnosis of vitamin B12 deficiency, prescription drug dementia or normal pressure hydrocephalus.

So, how big is this scandal? How many patients are involved? How many patients are currently sitting, or lying, in nursing homes, care homes, hospitals or the spare rooms of hard-pressed relatives because they have been misdiagnosed as suffering from Alzheimer's disease when, in reality, they could be treated quickly, easily and cheaply?

Officially, the figures show that around two thirds of dementia cases are caused by Alzheimer's. That is, without a doubt, a massive exaggeration. My professional estimate is that at least half of the patients diagnosed as having Alzheimer's are actually suffering from something quite different with prescription drug confusion, vitamin B12 shortage and normal pressure hydrocephalus being the three top diagnoses which are missed.

It is difficult to think of a bigger scandal in modern medicine.

Alzheimer's should be the very last diagnosis made when a patient is showing signs of dementia. It should not be the first diagnosis and it should certainly never be the default diagnosis.

Around the world there are millions of patients who are alleged to have incurable Alzheimer's disease but who are curable.

That's one scandal.

The other scandal is that no one in the medical profession or the media cares.

I doubt if anyone from the medical establishment, the big charities or the drug industry will be willing to debate this issue with me on television or radio.

They operate on the basis that if they ignore me then the facts will be ignored. And, sadly, no one in the establishment will take any notice of this book – even though the information I provide could change the lives of hundreds of thousands of patients. I have made many accurate predictions and judgements on medical matters over the years (there is a list on my main website www.vernoncoleman.com) but since my first two books (*The Medicine Men* and *Paper Doctors*) were published I have been ostracised, demonised and lied about by the drug company controlled medical establishment. My short book on normal pressure hydrocephalus was completely ignored by the media. Several experienced, journalists became excited by the book, and agreed that the misdiagnosis of the disease was a scandal. But their editors always quashed attempts to write about the scandal.

My conclusion is that anyone with dementia should be properly investigated for vitamin B12 deficiency or normal pressure hydrocephalus because, apart from dementia and confusion caused by prescription drugs, they are the commonest cause of dementia which are easily and permanently curable.

If the patient is shown not to have NPH or vitamin B12 deficiency and they are not taking regular doses of tranquillisers, sedatives and sleeping tablets, then, and only then, should doctors investigate the possibility that they might have Alzheimer's.

Chapter Two

How Critical Doctors Are Silenced

You would be forgiven for thinking I am exaggerating the power of the pharmaceutical industry, so let me tell you a true story which illustrates the power of the industry and which illustrates just how the pharmaceutical industry controls medical thinking.

A few years ago, I was invited to speak at an important conference in London.

The conference was, I was told, intended to tackle the subject of medication errors and adverse reactions to prescribed drugs. The company organising the conference was called PasTest.

'For over thirty years, PasTest has been providing medical education to professionals within the NHS,' they told me. 'Building on our commitment to quality in medical and healthcare education, PasTest is creating a range of healthcare events which focus on the professional development of clinicians and managers who are working together to deliver healthcare services for the UK. Our aim is to provide a means for those who are in a position to improve services on both national and regional levels. The topics covered by our conferences are embraced within policy, best practice, case study, clinical management and evidence based practice. PasTest endeavours to source the best speakers who will engage audiences with balanced, relevant and thought provoking programmes. PasTest has proven in the past that by using thorough investigative research and keeping up-to-date with advances in healthcare and medical practice, a premium educational event can be achieved.'

Goody, I thought.

Iatrogenesis (doctor induced disease) is something of a speciality of mine. I have written numerous books and articles on the subject. My campaigns have resulted in more drugs being banned or controlled than anyone else's. A previous Government admitted that they had taken action on prescription drug control because of my articles.

The conference organisers offered to pay me £1,500 plus £500 in expenses for two hours of my time. In addition to speaking at the conference, they wanted me to help them decide on the final programme.

I thought the conference was an important one and would give me a good opportunity to tell NHS staff the truth. I signed a contract, and PasTest duly wrote to confirm my appointment as a consultant and speaker for the PasTest Conference Division.

And then there was silence. My office repeatedly asked for details of when and where the conference was being held.

Silence.

Eventually, a programme for the event appeared on the internet. Curiously, my name was not on the list of speakers.

Here is part of the blurb promoting the conference:

'Against a background of increasing media coverage into the number of UK patients who are either becoming ill or dying due to adverse reactions to medication, our conference aims to explain the current strategies to avoid Adverse Drug reactions and what can be done to educate patients.'

Putting the blame on patients for problems caused by prescription drugs is brilliant. Most drug related problems are caused by the stupidity of doctors not the ignorance of patients. If the aim is to educate patients on how best to avoid prescription drug problems, the advice would be simple: 'Don't trust doctors. They are, by and large, a bunch of incompetent buffoons who do what they are told to do by drug company representatives.'

The promotion for the conference claimed that 'errors in medication...account for 4% of hospital bed capacity.' And that prescription drug problems 'reportedly kill up to 10,000 people a year in the UK'.

As I would have shown (had I not been banned from the conference) these figures were absurdly low. I had already published evidence showing that one in six hospital beds was occupied by patients who had been made ill by doctors. And there was, and is, plenty of evidence showing that doctors are now one of the top three causes of sickness and death (alongside cancer and circulatory disorders such as heart disease and stroke).

The list of speakers included a variety of people I had never heard of including one speaker representing The Association of the British Pharmaceutical Industry and another representing the Medicines and Healthcare Products Regulatory Agency.

Delegates representing the NHS were expected to pay £250 plus VAT (£293.75) to attend the event. Delegates whose Trust would be funding the cost were asked to apply for a Health Authority Approval form.

The NHS is paying to send delegates to a conference where someone representing the drug industry will speak to them on drug safety. But I'm banned. No longer allowed to speak. The truth has been uninvited.

So why am I now apparently banned from this conference?

This is what Simon Levy of PasTest said when we asked them: 'certain parties felt that he (Vernon Coleman) was too controversial to speak and as a result would not attend.'

Could that, I wonder, be the drug industry?

Is the drug industry now deciding whom they will allow to speak to doctors and NHS staff on the problems caused by prescription drugs?

If I was banned at the behest of the drug industry, do NHS bosses know that people attending the PasTest conference will only hear speakers approved by the drug industry?

If I was banned at the behest of the medical profession, why are doctors frightened of the truth? (If they think my views are wrong they would surely be happy for me to appear so that they could counter my arguments.)

I could not, of course, be banned by the NHS itself. Why would the NHS not want its employees to know the truth about drug related problems?

Why are people who had me banned so frightened of what I would say? It can surely only be because they know that I would have caused embarrassment by telling the truth.

PasTest offered me a fee of £1,500 to speak at this conference. Because we had a contract they have now paid me NOT to turn up. I used the money to buy advertisements for my book *How To Stop Your Doctor Killing You*.

Details of the ban were sent to every national and major local newspaper in Britain. None reported it.

I am by no means the only doctor to have found him or herself silenced in some way by the medical establishment. Every doctor I know of who has openly questioned vaccination has been persecuted and/or struck off the medical register.

Does that sound unlikely? Does my own experience sound unlikely? I sometimes fear that my own experiences may make me sound as though I am exhibiting well-established signs of paranoia.

But consider what happened to J. Meirion Thomas, a former specialist cancer surgeon at The Royal Marsden Hospital in London.

Dr Thomas's troubles began when he wrote a newspaper article in which he commented that 'the GP service is hopelessly outmoded'. The article had been written in response to a report from the Care Quality Commission. He wrote the article because he wanted to help improve patient care. And at the age of 68, he rightly thought he had experience which made his views worthwhile.

Nothing too controversial in that, you might think.

But the authorities thought otherwise. The medical establishment does not approve of doctors trying to improve things. And it does not approve of criticism – however valuable or well intended.

Here is what happened to Dr Thomas (a widely respected surgeon with many years of experience) immediately after the publication of his article:

1) He received a letter (which he describes as 'aggressive') from the Imperial College, where he was Professor of Surgical Oncology. The letter demanded that he immediately sever all relations with the college.

2) A petition was started to have him struck off the medical register by the General Medical Council.

3) He received a message from The Royal Marsden Hospital where he worked as a specialist cancer surgeon. He was summoned to a meeting where he was told he had brought the hospital into disrepute and would not be allowed to attend until further notice. He was forced to take 'authorised leave' from his work.

4) The chief executive of the The Royal Marsden Hospital received a complaint from the Professor of General Practice at Imperial College. Dr Thomas reports that 'this included a financial threat, querying why GPs should be expected to refer patients to The Royal Marsden Hospital when there are many others in London with which they had very good working relationships with the staff.'

5) Dr Thomas was then told that his Lifetime Achievement Award for 31 years of service at The Royal Marsden Hospital (due to be presented at a ceremony the following evening) was to be withdrawn.

6) He was eventually told he could return to work if he signed a document agreeing not to write any more articles unless he showed them to the chief executive in advance so that she could make sure they wouldn't harm the hospital's reputation.

All that happened because Dr Thomas dared to write one article about general practice.

The tragedy is that this sad story is not, I fear, in any way exceptional. It is, rather, the norm. Whistle blowers, truth-tellers and critics are not welcomed by the medical establishment. The doctors who are seen on television and heard on the radio are, I fear, largely vetted or approved by the pharmaceutical industry and the medical establishment (the two are pretty well interchangeable) for their willingness to toe the official line. The same is true, to a slightly lesser extent, of doctors who write for or are quoted in newspapers and magazines. Doctors who speak up on behalf of patients, or who try to expose problems within medical practice, will be quickly silenced. (It is much more difficult for the establishment to suppress doctors who write books – though even this is possible in that doctors regarded as troublemakers will usually find it impossible to promote their books on radio or television and they will also have to expect that their books will not be reviewed.)

You can now imagine the problems I have had after writing several thousand articles and scores of books about medical practice! I have been censored, banned and the subject of numerous complaints. Today, the combined efforts of the pharmaceutical industry and the medical establishment mean that no one will interview me, review my books or print my articles.

(I am not complaining – merely reporting the way things are.)

It is hardly surprising that very few doctors dare to write anything critical of established medical practices – however damaging or dangerous they might be.

Chapter Three

The Power of Modern Charities

'No one survives a diagnosis of dementia.'

The quote is attributed to Hilary Evans, the chief executive of Alzheimer's Research UK.

Did she really say that?

I suppose she must have done.

But it is NOT true.

I repeat: it is NOT true.

The Alzheimer Industry (a convenient mixture of drug companies and charities) seems determined to ignore the facts, regardless of the unnecessary fear which is produced.

I worry a good deal about the charities which are supposedly devoted to helping patients with dementia. Some of them claim that dementia is incurable and there seems to me to be a deliberate tendency to use the words dementia and Alzheimer's as though they were interchangeable.

The media do exactly the same thing, and health reporters working for newspapers, radio and television seem determined to promote the false idea that dementia is the same as Alzheimer's and that once a diagnosis of dementia is made then there is no hope. Consensus journalism is enormously popular everywhere these days.

The problem is that the big charities are driven by the same force as the pharmaceutical industry: money.

I have long been an enthusiastic supporter of patients' associations – small groups set up to defend and protect the interests of patients with specific health problems. The associations provide support and information for patients and also campaign on their behalf. Back in the late 1960s and early 1970s, I compiled the first directory of patients' associations. In those days, most such groups were small and run by volunteers – usually from someone's kitchen table. Money was raised by organising coffee mornings and selling raffle tickets. Cash which couldn't be raised in this way came from the wallets and handbags of volunteer organisers. Private telephones were used and newsletters were put together with a cheap copier machine and a stapler. Most of these small organisations were run on a hand to mouth basis.

And then the drug companies realised that these associations could be useful to them in a number of ways. To begin with they realised that the associations gave them a way of contacting their customers directly (without going through the prescribing doctors) and later, as the volunteers started to do local newspaper interviews to raise awareness of the illness with which they were concerned (and the association they had formed), the drug companies realised that they had discovered an excellent way to influence public opinion. Occasionally, there would be a chance for national publicity on radio or television or in a newspaper or magazine looking for a human interest story. The patients' associations could provide patients and relatives prepared to talk about their disease to a wide public. Newly formed local radio stations and local television stations had an insatiable demand for people to talk about diseases, and the volunteers who had created patients' associations found themselves in a powerful position.

The laws in most countries mean that drug companies are not allowed to advertise prescription only products directly to patients. Advertisements can only be aimed at the doctors prescribing the drugs. (This is why so many medical journals can make so much money.) Slowly, the drug companies which produced the pharmaceutical products these patients were taking, realised that the patients' associations offered them a way to communicate directly with patients. Through the patients' associations they could promote new products, they could explain why their product was better than anyone else's and they could influence the public's understanding of the disease concerned. Most important of all, they could use the patients' associations to control and denigrate the drug industry's own critics – whether the critics were alternative health practitioners or 'rogue' doctors drawing attention to side effects and other problems.

And so the drug companies started to approach the volunteers running small charities and to offer them financial help. It probably all seemed innocent and well-meaning. A dozen volunteers producing a newsletter for sufferers of a disease (let's call it Godwin's Disease because I know of no such disease) would be approached by a company (let's call it Islington International Pharmaceuticals because I know of no such company) which happened to be the manufacturer of a drug used in the treatment of Godwin's Disease. And the drug company would kindly offer to help.

'We all want to help patients,' the drug company would say. 'You are doing terrific work and we are a kindly, philanthropic organisation so please allow us to give you £500 to help pay for printing and posting your newsletter.'

The surprised volunteers would be enormously grateful. They would enthusiastically accept the £500 and it would make life a little easier.

Then, a few weeks later, when the £500 had gone, the drug company would come back and offer a larger sum.

'We think we can help more,' they would say. 'We would like to make a donation of £5,000. In return we would be pleased if you would put our logo onto your newsletter and your leaflets. This will enable us to tell the board of directors that our donation is advertising and is therefore justified.'

The volunteers would happily accept the £5,000.

And they would be hooked.

Before long, the volunteers would be working out of smart offices in the nearest town. Two or three of them would be paying themselves salaries, pension payments and expenses. And the drug company money would be essential and expected. The small charity would not be able to exist in its new form without the big cheques from Islington International Pharmaceuticals. The days of putting together a newsletter on the kitchen table would be forgotten. Sadly, the days of honesty and integrity would also be gone. The charity (for by now the volunteers would have doubtless been able to afford to register their association as a proper charity) would no longer rely on those little coffee mornings and those efforts to sell raffle tickets for a bottle of cheap wine.

This now happens all the time.

The sums involved can be quite large. And once the charity is hooked then the game is over. The drug company owns the charity and has a valuable mouthpiece.

'One or two people are criticising our bestselling product,' the drug company will say to one of the charity's employees. 'This is unreasonable and unfair and we know that support from you would help counteract the criticism.'

'What can we do to help?' will be the natural response.

'Our publicity department has contacted a few television and radio people and they would love to talk to you about appearing on their programmes. They will, of course, pay you a fee and provide you with a hotel and also pay your expenses.'

And so the charity employee would go on television and radio and enjoy the fame and the little bit of (personal) money, and they would duly say whatever it was that the drug company wanted them to say. 'Why not? We're all working together, aren't we?'

Many of the big charities now have very well paid executives and, of course, as they get bigger there is a risk that charities become 'corporate'. They end up with huge administrative staffs. They pay their executives six figure salaries – with massive expense accounts and pensions.

I know of well-known charities which spend less than a quarter of their income on the cause for which they are supposed to exist. Most of their income goes on salaries and administration. They long ago lost sight of the aims which kept them sat around the kitchen table. Actually, those people have long since gone; pushed aside by the professionals.

And some of these highly paid charity executives know damned well that they would have a job finding similarly well-paid employment outside the charity sector.

So, the charity's employees find that their aims are aligned with those of their sponsoring drug companies. And they certainly don't have an incentive to see anyone find a cure for 'their' disease. Once a cure has been found, there will be no need for a campaigning charity and the drug company's profits will collapse.

Much the same thing sort of happens in the world of animal rights.

Years ago I talked to someone working for an animal rights group and spoke with enthusiasm about putting an end to a particular variety of animal cruelty.

'Oh we don't actually want it to stop,' he told me, shamelessly. 'If it stops then we'll be out of work.'

And, of course, as they get bigger and richer so charities find that they need to keep growing; they need to acquire more members and more support and more donations. Naturally, the bigger they get the more the drug companies like it.

I have on my desk a leaflet entitled 'Worried about your memory?' It is a leaflet about dementia. But the only cause of dementia which is mentioned is Alzheimer's disease. The clear assumption is that if a patient is suffering from memory loss then they are probably suffering from Alzheimer's disease. The leaflet, inevitably, contains an address and a website for the Alzheimer's Society. And there is a telephone number for the Alzheimer's Society's National Dementia Helpline. At the bottom of the leaflet there is a slogan 'Leading the fight against dementia. Alzheimer's Society'.

And there is also a drug company logo announcing that the production of the leaflet has been supported by Lilly.

Eli Lilly is a drug company which claims it has been a global leader in the fight against Alzheimer's disease for nearly 30 years. Its products include 'seven investigational compounds to treat Alzheimer's and two diagnostics to help better diagnose it'.

I wouldn't expect Lilly to point out that there are many causes of memory loss other than Alzheimer's disease.

And, sadly, nor would I expect the Alzheimer's Society to point out that there are many other causes of memory loss.

Off the top of my head I can think of alcoholism, thyroid, kidney and liver disorders, normal pressure hydrocephalus, tumours, strokes, infections and head injury. And, of course, vitamin B12 deficiency and prescription drug side effects are almost certainly commoner causes of memory loss and confusion than Alzheimer's disease.

And when I put 'memory loss' into the Google search engine, the first item which appeared was 'Memory loss and dementia – Alzheimer's Society'. I suppose the charity pays to dominate the search but it is, of course, misleading patients by associating memory loss and dementia with a single, dramatically over-diagnosed disease.

I think this business of corralling patients in this way is dishonest, immoral, unethical and immensely harmful.

Chapter Four

The NHS Misleads

It isn't just charities which mislead about dementia.

In the UK, the NHS is still distributing inaccurate information about dementia. For example, I have on my desk a leaflet published by something called Public Health England in conjunction with the Alzheimer's Society and Alzheimer's Research UK. The leaflet states categorically that dementia cannot be cured.

This is a lie. It is a dangerous, manipulative, commercially directed, evil lie.

I reckon that at least half of all the individuals diagnosed with dementia could be cured in a week or two.

Dementia which is caused by normal pressure hydrocephalus (one of the commonest causes) can be cured with a simple operation. Dementia caused by vitamin B12 deficiency (almost certainly much commoner than dementia caused by Alzheimer's disease) can be cured with a course of injections.

And vast numbers of patients with so-called dementia could be cured simply by taking them off their tranquillisers and sleeping tablets. The tablets cause confusion, dementia is diagnosed (usually Alzheimer's) and so more tablets are prescribed. It is this problem which explains why the incidence of dementia appears to be increasing so rapidly.

My guess is that around half of all patients who have been diagnosed as having dementia are curable within a week.

(Anyone stopping pills of any kind should do so under medical supervision in order to supervise the withdrawal period – which can be difficult.)

Why does no one care about the truth about dementia? Why are these truths suppressed? Why cannot they even be debated?

Sadly, the answer is simple. The NHS, the medical profession and the dementia charities only tell people what the drug industry wants them to tell them.

The medical establishment was bought long ago by the pharmaceutical giants.

Chapter Five

Medical Journals – Corrupt and Misleading

The dishonesty and ruthlessness of the pharmaceutical industry would be of no account were the medical profession not ready and willing to be corrupted.

But you don't have to look far to see just how the profession has been corrupted by drug company money.

Drug company money and influence is everywhere. Doctors receive free journals paid for by drug companies. Doctors are taken out to lunch and dinner by drug companies. Medical meetings are sponsored by drug companies (and described as post graduate education). Doctors are paid huge fees to perform small 'research' tasks which could more fairly be described as 'marketing'. And doctors conducting research projects are given grants by drug companies. (Very little medical research takes place that is not funded by drug companies. It is for this reason that most of the research conducted promotes products – rather than questioning their value. And so, as far as I am aware, no research has ever been done to question the value of vaccinations.)

Not long ago an eminent American doctor, Dr Dean Ornish, devised a safe, effective treatment programme for heart disease that depended upon diet, exercise and relaxation. However, Dr Ornish was denied funds by the American government and the American Heart Association, and Dr Ornish was quoted as having been told that drugs are essential in the treatment of heart disease because it is impossible to persuade people to change their drug taking habits.

I sometimes feel that the medical establishment is single-minded in its devotion to opposing real progress and suppressing original thought.

Most medical journals exist mainly as marketing tools for the pharmaceutical industry. Most of the papers which are published are written by doctors who have at some stage in their careers received money or goods from drug companies. Some of the papers published in reputable sounding journals are published only because a drug company with a product to sell has paid the journal to publish a particular paper because it helps to promote a new product. It has been well established that drug companies will, when it is commercially appropriate, suppress the publication of scientific papers which are considered commercially harmful.

Even the most reputable journals are not beyond criticism.

So, for example, consider the medical journal *The Lancet*. There are hundreds of medical journals in existence but *The Lancet* has been around a long time, is venerated within the profession and is probably no better or worse than the rest. I am sure that *The Lancet* would not agree to suppress an unsuitable paper or publish a paper which was unsound. And, as with most journals, authors of papers must these days state if they have any financial connection with a drug company related to their area of research.

But I am still sceptical about the attitude of all medical journals. I know of no medical journal for example, which would give this book half an inch of review space. My experience is that issues which are unpopular with the drug companies (the usefulness of vivisection or the questioning of the value and safety of vaccination for example) are ignored by all medical journals.

Medical journalists writing for popular papers often quote articles which have appeared in *The Lancet* but it is, I think, worth pointing out that *The Lancet* is a commercial journal which charges a good deal of money for advertising. The latest circulation figures for the weekly magazine show that back in 2007 it sold 29,103 copies and yet despite this relatively modest circulation, a full page advert in *The Lancet* can cost up to £10,800 (though it will be considerably more than that if you want to buy the back cover). I can only offer the circulation rate for 2007 because, even in 2019, that was the only figure I could find on *The Lancet's* website.

Now compare that advertising rate with a magazine that, it is fair to assume, does not take a good deal of drug company advertising. At random I picked a magazine called *Model Rail Magazine*. It has a circulation of 28,337. And the most expensive page rate for a full page is £900.

So, an advert in *The Lancet* costs more than ten times as much as an advert in *Model Rail Magazine*.

And who buys the advertising in *The Lancet*?

Well, if you guessed that most of it was paid for by drug companies then you probably would not be far off the mark.

And who makes vaccines?

Well, drug companies of course.

Am I being unfair in fearing that there could be a conflict of interest here? I don't think so.

I would have more respect for *The Lancet* (and its point of view) if the magazine refused all drug company advertising and relied entirely on subscription fees. It is worth noting that a subscription to *The Lancet* costs £163 whereas a subscription to *Model Rail Magazine* costs £51. Moreover, I doubt if *The Lancet* pays much if anything to its contributors whereas *Model Rail Magazine* doubtless has quite a substantial editorial cost.

This astonishing discrepancy in advertising rates is commonplace within the world of medical publishing. There are thousands of medical journals and magazines in existence around the world and many of them are hugely profitable. Drug companies use their journal advertising to promote drugs directly to the doctors with the prescription pads.

The drug companies use charities to indoctrinate patients and they use medical journals to indoctrinate doctors.

Part Two: The Causes of Dementia

Chapter One

Prescription Drugs

Drugs, depression and illness can all mimic the symptoms of dementia and, therefore, the modern default diagnosis of Alzheimer's disease.

This is not a new discovery.

When, in 2003, my wife and I wrote a book entitled *How To Conquer Health Problems Between Ages 50 and 120*, we made it clear that prescription drugs were a common cause of dementia. Here is what we said: 'It is possible that prescription drugs, not Alzheimer's, are the commonest cause of dementia. It is likely that half of all cases of alleged dementia could be cured simply by stopping unnecessary prescription drug use. Sedatives, hypnotics, anxiolytics and anti-depressants are the commonest cause of problems, with benzodiazepine tranquillisers and sleeping tablets such as Valium, Mogadon and Ativan probably being some of the commonest culprits.'

Since we wrote that paragraph in 2003, the situation has deteriorated and I am now quite certain that prescription drugs – not Alzheimer's – are the commonest cause of dementia.

The significance of this can best be illustrated by pointing out that it is likely that half of all cases of alleged dementia could be cured simply by stopping unnecessary prescription drug use.

In the UK alone there are several million patients regularly taking tranquillisers or anti-depressants. Many have been taking the drugs for months if not for years; often obtaining their supplies by applying for repeat prescriptions. There are thousands of patients around who take these drugs every day but who have not seen a doctor for years. In my book *The Benzos Story*, I pointed out that many patients had been taking benzodiazepines for over ten years without ever seeing a doctor. What most of these patients probably don't realise is that the list of side effects for these drugs is long and rather alarming and there is no doubt whatsoever that patients who take these drugs can develop all the signs and symptoms of dementia.

The evidence for this has been available for nearly half a century.

Here is a summary of some of the evidence showing the problems which can occur with benzodiazepine drugs.

In 1968, a paper published in the *Journal of the American Medical Association*, showed that benzodiazepines can cause depression so severe that suicidal thoughts occurred.

In 1972, a letter appeared in the *British Medical Journal* in which two specialists from Newcastle General Hospital pointed out that nitrazepam was particularly unsuitable for older patients. It was reported elsewhere that a 75-year-old woman became confused, incontinent and unable to walk or speak clearly after taking one 5mg tablet of nitrazepam every night for a year or so.

In 1972, a paper published in the *American Journal of Psychiatry* by Lt Cdr Richard C.W. Hall and Joy R Joffe MD, showed how patients who had taken diazepam had suffered from apprehension, insomnia, depression and tremulousness.

In 1979, a psychiatrist in Holland described how patients who had taken a benzodiazepine had developed severe anxiety and intolerable psychological changes.

In 1982, a British professor of psychopharmacology, Malcolm Lader reported on evidence showing that patients who had taken diazepam for some years had damaged brains.

In 1982, the *Scandinavian Journal of Psychology* published a paper entitled 'Amnesic Effects of Diazepam: Drug dependence explained by state dependent learning'. The paper, written by Hans Henrik Jensen and Jens Christian Poulsen, showed that patients who take diazepam won't be able to remember things they learned while taking the drug – unless they take it again.

In the period from January 1964 to February 1982, the Committee on Safety of Medicines in London received reports of well over 100 different side effects related to diazepam alone. The side effects included visual disturbances, headaches, confusion and dizziness.

There is no doubt that patients who have been taking benzodiazepine tranquillisers for more than a week or two are quite likely to develop symptoms which could be misdiagnosed as dementia.

Similarly, it is also likely that patients who have been prescribed sleeping tablets or anti-depressants for more than a week or two might easily develop symptoms of confusion and so on which could easily be mistaken for dementia.

(In 1988, the British Government took action to warn doctors about the dangerous of benzodiazepines. The Government admitted that they had taken action because of my articles on the subject. At that time I warned that if doctors were reluctant to prescribe benzodiazepines, the drug companies would simply encourage doctors to use powerful anti-depressants instead. Knowing something of how the drug industry works this was not a particularly difficult prediction to make. This is, of course, exactly what happened. Doctors now prescribe anti-depressants at the slightest indication of unhappiness or discontent. My book describing the battle to control the prescribing of benzodiazepines is described in *The Benzos Story: 1960-1980s.*)

The problems start when the patient who has drug-induced dementia is given the default diagnosis of Alzheimer's disease – this is, after all, the default diagnosis for bewildered and confused patients.

There is better than even chance that the doctor will increase the dose of the benzodiazepine tranquilliser to help sedate and calm the troubled patient.

The result, of course, will be that the patient deteriorates still further and the doctor can smugly claim that his diagnosis was clearly the correct one.

Drugs advertised as alleviating the symptoms of Alzheimer's disease will then be prescribed and probably added to the mixture.

Chapter Two

Inadequate Vitamin B12

Let me start this chapter with two certainties.

First, it is reliably estimated that between 3% and 5% of the population are deficient in vitamin B12. Some experts put the figure as high as 10% and it is suggested that at least a fifth of all those over the age of 60 have low vitamin B12. The certainty is that vitamin B12 deficiency is an epidemic.

Second, it is an established fact that individuals who are deficient in vitamin B12 are likely to suffer from a wide range of symptoms with dementia being one of the most significant of those symptoms.

So, around the world, how many of the many millions said to be suffering from Alzheimer's disease are in reality simply vitamin B12 deficient and could be cured with a short course of injections?

Your guess is as good as mine but we have to be talking about several hundred thousand patients in the UK alone. I'd suspect that the real figure is around 500,000.

If I am right that means that Alzheimer's disease is nowhere near as common as it is said to be and that half a million patients with Alzheimer's disease could have been cured with a simple two week course of injections.

The symptoms produced by vitamin B12 deficiency are many and varied. Vitamin B12 is absolutely essential for the human body to function properly. (There is an appendix at the back of this book in which I have listed some of the symptoms most commonly associated with vitamin B12 deficiency.)

The symptoms I am most concerned with in this book are obviously those which relate to mental issues – specifically those which could be diagnosed as dementia.

So, why is vitamin B12 deficiency being overlooked?

That's simple.

There are three simple reasons and one underlying and more complicated reason.

First, most doctors don't bother to test for vitamin B12 deficiency. There is a cheap and simple blood test available but doctors don't usually take the trouble to order it. If you don't test for vitamin B12 deficiency you won't ever find it.

Second, normal figures vary from laboratory to laboratory. This is lunacy, of course. But it's what happens. If samples of your blood are sent to two laboratories the chances are that the acceptable 'normal' figures will be different.

Third, the laboratories which do the blood tests usually give the wrong 'normal' result figures. They have been doing this for years. If a doctor sends a blood sample to a laboratory he will probably be told that a patient is only deficient in vitamin B12 if the result shows a reading of under 180 or so. And that is just plain wrong. It has been reliably established that a patient who has a blood reading of under 350-400 is almost certainly dangerously short of vitamin B12. And the shortage can be remedied with a few very cheap injections of vitamin B12.

When a patient's vitamin B12 level is down below 350, they will be quite ill. Indeed, at that point a patient will be showing severe signs of deficiency. But the patient won't be treated until their vitamin B12 level is down below 180.

In its 'Cobalamin and Folate Guidelines', the British Committee for Standards in Haematology says: 'The clinical picture is the most important factor in assessing the significance of test results assessing cobalamin status since there is no 'gold standard' test to define deficiency'.

Many experts now seem to think that symptoms rather than blood levels should be the deciding factor in deciding treatment. A study of the literature shows a clear conclusion that long-term blood levels probably need to be at least 350-400 and that the standard lab figures for vitamin B12 deficiency are far too low.

An article in the *British Journal of Haematology* in 2014 ('Guidelines for the diagnosis and treatment of cobalamin and folate disorders') suggests that doctors should consider treating patients who have vitamin B12 levels in the 'low-normal' range rather than the lower figures still being recommended by laboratories.

My conclusion is that it is a tragedy that laboratories persist in recommending 180 as a trigger point for treatment.

And since local laboratories and GPs like to look at test results before planning treatment (it makes them feel like scientists and gives them something to hold onto when they contemplate the possibility of legal action for malpractice), all the patients whose vitamin B12 levels are shown to be above 180 will be told that they are not short of vitamin B12 but have something else wrong with them.

(The precise figure varies from country to country and, within the NHS, from one district to another. As though to complicate and confuse things still further, different laboratories measure vitamin B12 in different ways. Here, I have quoted figures for pg/ml but vitamin B12 is also measured in pmol/L and ng/L. To avoid all these complications I have chosen the most common figure – which is 180 pg/ml.)

It is not surprising that one recent survey showed that 14% of the patients who were eventually diagnosed with symptoms caused by vitamin B12 deficiency waited more than ten years for the diagnosis to be made. During that decade or more they suffered constantly from mental and physical symptoms and their conditions deteriorated steadily.

And it is not surprising that in a paper published in the *British Journal of Haematology*, 2014 and entitled 'Guidelines for the diagnosis and treatment and cobalamin and folate disorders' the authors (V. Devalia, M. Hamilton and A. Molloy) concluded: 'We suggest that physicians should consider treating patients who show symptoms but have vitamin B12 levels…in the low-normal range up to approximately 300 pmol/l…'.

That seems to be a decent compromise. The advice seems to me to be: 'since our recommended blood levels are so useless we suggest that you ignore them and pretty much rely on how the patient feels'.

However, it doesn't seem as though many doctors know any of this and so older patients who are short of vitamin B12, and who are showing mental signs of being deficient in vitamin B12, are usually just diagnosed as suffering from dementia.

And, of course, the medical default diagnosis for dementia is Alzheimer's disease.

So the patient gets put into a long stay residential home and is given regular and expensive doses of drugs which won't do much (if any) good but which are much more profitable than a course of vitamin B12 injections.

Meanwhile, the younger patients who are short of vitamin B12 and who are showing physical signs such as muscle weakness and instability, and probably some mental signs too, will be diagnosed as suffering from multiple sclerosis because that is the default diagnosis for these symptoms in patients under 60 years of age.

And, like Alzheimer's disease, there is no specific test for multiple sclerosis. Isn't that just wonderfully convenient?

And these patients, now labelled as suffering from multiple sclerosis, will either struggle on at home or they will be put into some sort of residential care. And wherever they are they will be prescribed regular and expensive drugs which probably won't make much if any difference to their condition but which will be hugely profitable for the companies which make them.

(As an aside, is it impossible that all multiple sclerosis patients might be suffering from undiagnosed vitamin B12 deficiency? Both disorders have problems caused by demyelination and the symptoms involved with multiple sclerosis and vitamin B12 deficiency are identical.)

So, that's how medicine works these days.

This isn't going to change until a patient sues a laboratory and complains that their misleading reading resulted in a good deal of unnecessary mental and physical suffering.

And there is no doubt that mental and physical suffering occurs.

When a patient's blood level of vitamin B12 is below 350, their body will already be starting to show signs of damage. And the damage will be serious. Around three quarters of patients with low vitamin B12 will suffer neurological symptoms, for vitamin B12 deficiency causes megaloblastic anaemia and demyelinating disease. (It is the demyelination which means that vitamin B12 shortage leads to symptoms which are identical to those seen with multiple sclerosis.)

If this sounds too awful to be true let me provide you with some evidence.

The New England Journal of Medicine reported in 2013 that patients with B12 deficiency develop demyelinating disease (hence the reason why so many patients are diagnosed as suffering from MS) and that patients frequently complain of muscle weakness, paraesthesia and gait problems.

The Journal of Clinical Psychiatry reported in 2009 that patients who are low in vitamin B12 suffer from neuropsychiatric disorders as well as neuropathy. Specifically listed problems include depression, dementia, auditory hallucinations, suicidal thoughts, mental impairment and psychosis.

Numerous papers in reputable medical journals have established a clear link between vitamin B12 deficiency and psychosis with many reporting that patients with low vitamin B12 may suffer from suicidal thoughts and hallucinations and then be wrongly diagnosed and treated as suffering from schizophrenia.

That's the bad news.

The good news, of course, is that if patients are given vitamin B12 (usually by a simple, cheap injection) they will get better quickly and their symptoms will be reversed. The injections are given regularly until there is clear improvement in the patient's symptoms and blood levels need to be monitored regularly.

So, why do doctors not do this simple test? Why are laboratories using the wrong measurements? Why are so many patients being mistreated?

That, I am afraid, takes us to the underlying, complicated reason.

The fact is that the drug companies which control the medical establishment (and which also control much postgraduate medical education and, through their advertising budgets, keep the medical journals alive) know that there is very little profit to be made out of identifying and treating vitamin B12 deficiency. Vitamin supplements and high dose injections are not patented and so they are very cheap. No one makes much money out of them.

I cannot overstress the fact that for many years now the pharmaceutical industry has pretty well owned the medical profession; it has certainly taken out a long lease on the medical establishment. The drug companies control how doctors practice and, most important of all, they control the way that doctors think.

If doctors do not routinely test their patients for vitamin B12 deficiency (and they do not) then a large number of patients who have physical and mental symptoms caused by a shortage of vitamin B12 will be diagnosed as suffering from other conditions – most commonly and most notably Alzheimer's disease and multiple sclerosis.

Multiple sclerosis is, like Alzheimer's disease, a disorder for which there is no specific test. It is a diagnosis which ought to be made when all other possibilities have been discounted.

But, these are profitable diseases. Patients with both disorders tend to live a long time. These are truly chronic disorders. And there are drugs available (very expensive drugs) which appear to provide some relief. The drugs don't cure the disease. The chronic nature of the disease means that patients suffer for years (sometimes for decades). Their symptoms and signs gradually get worse. But the chronic nature of their disease also means that the drug companies make enormous profits out of them.

And so multiple sclerosis is a default diagnosis for thousands of patients – in just the same way that Alzheimer's disease is a default diagnosis for patients with dementia.

You will not be surprised to learn that, as with Alzheimer's disease, multiple sclerosis is a disease which has attracted some large charities. And those charities receive a good deal of money from drug companies.

It is impossible to be precise but I would guess that probably half the patients who have been diagnosed as suffering from multiple sclerosis could have been cured if their vitamin B12 levels had been assessed and they had been treated with vitamin B12 injections. I can't think of a safer medicine with which to treat people. Vitamin B12 is water soluble and any excess is merely excreted in the urine. I haven't been able to find any evidence of anyone ever dying (or becoming seriously ill) as a result of treatment with vitamin B12. It is that rarest and most wonderful of treatments: a cheap and safe drug.

As I mentioned at the start of this chapter, vitamin B12 deficiency is very common. It affects millions of people. The symptoms of vitamin B12 deficiency vary from patient to patient but include the following: fatigue; weakness, especially in arms and legs; sore tongue; nausea; appetite loss; weight loss; bleeding gums; numbness and tingling in hands and feet; difficulty in maintaining balance; pale lips; pale tongue; pale gums; yellow eyes and skin; shortness of breath; depression; confusion and dementia; headache; poor memory. The first obvious signs of B12 deficiency might be pins and needles or coldness in the hands and feet, fatigue and weakness, poor concentration or even psychosis.

There are many reasons for the deficiency.

Some patients cannot absorb the vitamin (either because of an absence of intrinsic factor in their stomachs or because their small intestines are damaged in some way and cannot absorb it) and some patients are deficient because their diets don't contain enough of the foods which contain vitamin B12. Since vitamin B12 deficiency is common in those who follow a vegan diet it is likely that the current fashion for veganism will increase the occurrence of vitamin B12 deficiency.

Instead of checking the vitamin B12 levels for all susceptible patients (and remember, at least one in five people over the age of 60 is likely to have a dangerously low level of vitamin B12 in their blood), doctors prefer to check cholesterol levels.

Checking cholesterol levels is now hugely popular (and is an industry in itself) and millions of patients who have levels regarded as high are being treated – most commonly with drugs called statins. The drug companies are making an absolute fortune out of drugs prescribed to control cholesterol levels.

There are a few problems with this policy.

First, the evidence showing that cholesterol levels are significant is rather wobbly. And there are a good many independent doctors who believe that cholesterol levels are pretty meaningless. There are even arguments about different types of cholesterol – good cholesterol and bad cholesterol.

Second, there is evidence showing that reducing cholesterol levels can be dangerous. Patients whose cholesterol levels are reduced can become ill. This information isn't new and it isn't hidden. Indeed I wrote about it in my book *How To Stop Your Doctor Killing You* which was first published in 1996.

Third, the drugs most commonly used to reduce cholesterol levels are the statins. And they can cause a number of problems. Once again I wrote about statins in *How To Stop Your Doctor Killing You* in 1996.

So, here is yet more evidence showing that doctors do tests that are likely to produce evidence which is helpful to drug companies – rather than doing tests to produce evidence which helps patients. The only certainty is that treating cholesterol levels is an enormously profitable business and quite a growth industry.

If doctors really cared about the health of their patients they would leave cholesterol alone and put their effort into testing for the amount of vitamin B12 in the blood.

Chapter Three

Normal Pressure Hydrocephalus

The diagnosis of normal pressure hydrocephalus is missed more than 80% of the time. Between 5% and 10% of patients diagnosed as suffering from Alzheimer's disease or dementia are in fact suffering from the curable disease idiopathic normal pressure hydrocephalus – which can be fairly easily treated with a simple operation.

The three symptoms of idiopathic normal pressure hydrocephalus are:

A tendency to fall a good deal. If an elderly patient falls a lot then a diagnosis of idiopathic normal pressure hydrocephalus must be considered.

Dementia.

Urinary incontinence.

Why do doctors continue to ignore normal pressure hydrocephalus and to suppress the evidence of its significance?

There are two reasons.

First, idiopathic normal pressure hydrocephalus can be treated and cured with a simple surgical operation. Drug companies make millions out of selling drugs for the treatment of Alzheimer's disease and if patients with idiopathic normal pressure hydrocephalus were properly diagnosed, the demand for their drugs would plummet. And profits would fall. Sadly, many charities now work hand in glove with drug companies and so they follow the company line.

Second, doctors in the UK are now paid a generous fee whenever they make a diagnosis of Alzheimer's disease. But they do not get paid when they make a diagnosis of normal pressure hydrocephalus. Doctors have a financial interest in over-diagnosing Alzheimer's disease.

The result is that countless millions of patients with idiopathic normal pressure hydrocephalus have been diagnosed as suffering from Alzheimer's disease. They have been given drugs and abandoned. They have been left to die when they could have been treated and cured.

The truth is that the medical establishment is so influenced by the drug industry that it pays little attention to normal pressure hydrocephalus which is, as a result, under-researched, under-diagnosed and under-treated. There is almost certainly no disease affecting large numbers of people which is less understood. Within the medical profession it is known (when it is known at all) as the 'wet, wacky and wobbly disease' – more a childhood term of abuse than a phrase redolent with respect.

Organisations which specialise in caring for the elderly are often appallingly ignorant about the disease, as are health websites. I asked the questions on the internet, 'why are old people unstable?' and 'why do old people fall?' and none of the first several dozen responses mentioned 'normal pressure hydrocephalus'. In the UK, the NHS Choices website devotes less than 70 words to the disease and describes the condition as 'uncommon' which is manifest nonsense since it affects a vast number of patients and is (with vitamin B12 deficiency) the commonest treatable cause of major disability and mental incapacity among the elderly.

Researchers are not interested in investigating the disease because a cure is already available and, since there is no need for a 'wonder drug' there are not going to be any big, fat grants from drug companies. And doctors are not interested in diagnosing or treating the disease because it invariably involves older patients, and doctors are encouraged by governments (and much of society) not to take much interest in elderly patients. (Remember too, that the Government in the UK gives doctors a bonus every time they diagnose Alzheimer's disease. There is no bonus for diagnosing other causes of dementia.)

If you made a list of the 100 commonest, potentially fatal but most easily cured medical conditions which are most often mistakenly diagnosed as something else, then normal pressure hydrocephalus would be top of the list.

The only things we know for certain are that idiopathic normal pressure hydrocephalus is much commoner than is generally thought, produces devastating results, is usually mistaken for something else and it is treatable. Patients who have been stuck in bed or in wheelchairs can, after treatment, get up and walk. They can resume their lives; talking and enjoying work and hobbies. Patients who have been abandoned have their lives back. (See the case histories at the back of this book for examples of this statement).

So, what is normal pressure hydrocephalus?

Under normal circumstances the space between the brain and the skull is filled with cerebrospinal fluid; a substance which is produced within the spaces of the brain, circulates in and around the brain and is gradually reabsorbed. In normal circumstances, the fluid is produced in the same quantities as it is being reabsorbed. The cerebrospinal fluid, which also surrounds the spinal cord, is there primarily to protect the brain in case of injury.

In the condition known as normal pressure hydrocephalus, the fluid is not reabsorbed as fast as it is produced.

When there is too much fluid in and around the brain, the stuff accumulates in the ventricles – the spaces within the brain – and the brain is put under pressure, being pushed outwards. The result of this unusual pressure is that the brain is compressed and damaged in a variety of ways. The symptoms and signs of damage will depend upon the area of the brain affected. If the problem is not treated then the damage to the brain will be irreversible.

Logically, one might expect that with too much fluid in a confined space there would be an increase in fluid pressure. By definition this does not happen with normal pressure hydrocephalus. The intracranial pressure is normal and instead of putting up the pressure, the increased amount of fluid dilates the ventricular system. If a scan is done, the ventricles usually look dilated. However, even when patients have a magnetic resonance imaging (MRI) of the brain or computerised tomography (CT), the wrong diagnosis can still be made because doctors who are not aware of normal pressure hydrocephalus will probably assume not that the ventricles have become larger but that the brain has become smaller as a result of cerebral atrophy.

There are two types of normal pressure hydrocephalus – secondary and idiopathic. Secondary normal pressure hydrocephalus can be caused by a variety of external problems including a head injury, a tumour, an infection or a bleed. But idiopathic normal pressure hydrocephalus occurs with no underlying cause – it just happens.

Idiopathic normal pressure hydrocephalus, which was first described in 1965 by Hakim and Adams, does not appear to be any commoner in men than in women than in men, and there is not as yet any evidence showing whether it is particularly likely to affect any particular racial or ethnic groups. Although it can affect people of any age it does, however, seem to be most commonly seen among patients in their sixties or older and it is this which results in patients being so often misdiagnosed as suffering from Alzheimer's disease.

'There are no cures for many types of dementia. But there are some treatable forms of dementia, and normal pressure hydrocephalus is one of them,' said Ann Marie Flannery, a neurosurgeon at Women's and Children's Hospital in Lafayette, Louisiana, reported in *US News Health Care*.

The symptoms of idiopathic normal pressure hydrocephalus make it surprisingly easy to diagnose.

The initial, main symptom is often a curious, wide-legged, unsteady walk. The patient's feet seem to stick to the floor, and have to be dragged up in order to make the next step. Patients adopt a wide-legged gait in an attempt to make themselves more stable but they are, nevertheless, often unstable and may fall. Indeed, falling is a common problem with patients suffering from idiopathic normal pressure hydrocephalus, and in any elderly person who falls more than once or twice, the possible diagnosis of idiopathic normal pressure hydrocephalus should be placed quite high up on the list of possible causes.

Sadly, it is still the case that many leading health websites do not even mention normal pressure hydrocephalus as a possible cause of falls though since it is fairly common and treatable, the disorder should be listed towards the top of any such list, together with balance problems and drug side effects.

Since time is of the essence in diagnosing idiopathic normal pressure hydrocephalus, this disorder should always be considered very early on when a patient has fallen more than once or twice. Simply dismissing falls as 'an inevitable part of ageing', as some doctors are prone to do, is grossly irresponsible and unprofessional. Falling is not associated with any of the other common dementias, such as Alzheimer's disease.

The gait disturbance tends to get steadily worse as the amount of fluid increases and the ventricles within the brain expand. When the ventricles expand, they put pressure on the part of the nervous system which descends into the spinal cord.

In the early stages of normal pressure hydrocephalus, the gait disturbance will probably be mild and result in the patient being unsteady and having impaired balance, particularly when trying to walk up and down stairs or steps or even kerbs. The patient will probably also complain that their legs feel weak, though there will probably be no explanation for this.

As the disease progresses, so the patient's gait steadily gets worse. The patient will not lift their feet properly when walking and will walk very slowly. It is because of the gait disturbance that normal pressure hydrocephalus is often misdiagnosed as Parkinson's disease. The tendency to fall is so common in normal pressure hydrocephalus that it is, I think, reasonable to say that if a patient falls a good deal and suffers from some form of dementia then a diagnosis of idiopathic normal pressure hydrocephalus must be considered first of all.

In the final stages of the disease, patients may be unable to walk, then unable to stand and finally even unable turn over when lying in bed.

The second symptom is dementia, a chronic disorder of the mental processes which is caused by some brain disease or injury and which is characterised by mental disorder, personality changes and impaired reasoning. And this is why normal pressure hydrocephalus is so often misdiagnosed as Alzheimer's disease, or some other cause of dementia. The dementia in idiopathic normal pressure hydrocephalus usually involves the frontal lobe (because of the situation of the swelling ventricles within the brain) and patients will usually appear slow witted, forgetful and apathetic. There may be an absence of mood (patients are neither happy when they might be expected to be happy nor sad when sadness might be appropriate) and patients often have difficulty in speaking. The first sign of the dementia associated with this disease is often a curious difficulty in planning, organising or putting things in order. The patient may also have difficulty in paying attention and in thinking in an abstract way.

Patients may lose interest in daily activities, they forget names and things to be done, they have difficulty in dealing with routine tasks and their short-term memory may be poor. (One sufferer complained that he could no longer read a book because when he got to page 10 he could not remember what had happened on page 1.)

Although this symptom is usually placed second chronologically, it may be noticeable much earlier in some patients. I suspect that the reason the mental problems are not recognised or recorded, may often be because relatives and friends don't know what to look for, don't register subtle changes as being indicative of any underlying pathology and may dismiss changes as being simply consequences of 'old age'.

It is important to remember that dementia is not a disease but a consequence of some underlying disease. And it is vital to remember that although the dementia associated with normal pressure hydrocephalus may appear similar, in superficial terms, to the dementia associated with Alzheimer's disease, the two underlying disorders are quite different entities. There is, sadly, no cure for Alzheimer's disease at the moment but there is a remarkably effective and relatively simple cure available for normal pressure hydrocephalus. To describe normal pressure hydrocephalus as a variation of Alzheimer's disease (as I have seen done) is as nonsensical as describing heart disease as a type of cancer.

The final symptom to occur is often urinary incontinence.

Patients tend to have an increased sense of urgency (they suddenly need to urinate) but in the later stages, as the frontal lobe damage increases, they become indifferent to the consequences and genuine urinary incontinence may result. In some cases the urinary incontinence may occur quite early on in the disease. Some patients also develop faecal incontinence.

Mainstream medical textbooks do not include headache as a significant symptom in this condition but it can occur and it seems perfectly reasonable that it should do so. After all, the brain is being compressed and squashed against the skull and the eyes are under constant pressure. It would be rather unlikely if patients with this condition did not have, at the very least, an uncomfortable feeling in their heads.

Patients may also have difficulty in focussing their eyes and occasionally, towards the end of the patient's life, the eyes may bulge as the pressure of fluid builds up.

Whatever symptoms may occur they tend to progress with time, sometimes slowly and sometimes quite quickly. Careful questioning of the patient suggests that symptoms may have been present for months or even years before a doctor was consulted. By then the patient may have, to a certain extent, become accustomed to their disability and the chances are high that they themselves will have learned to regard the difficulty in walking, the slowness of thought or the incontinence as an inevitable consequence of ageing. In many cases it is only when there is a critical loss of function, or a disability which dramatically affects the patient's independence, which leads to the patient seeking medical advice. At that point, the chances are high that the only solution on offer will be a default diagnosis of Alzheimer's disease, a bed in a nursing home or hospice or a suggestion that a relative should take over and provide accommodation and care.

The symptoms associated with normal pressure hydrocephalus do vary a good deal. The one constant factor seems to be the delay in making the diagnosis. Time and time again patients and relatives will report that it took years for an accurate diagnosis to be made and that even then it was only after the patient had seen a good many doctors. The evidence now suggests that in 80% of patients the correct diagnosis is never made.

So, how common is idiopathic normal pressure hydrocephalus?

Idiopathic normal pressure hydrocephalus has been so little investigated that it is difficult to be certain how common it really is but there are three ways to tackle this vital question. All these methods make it very clear that idiopathic normal pressure hydrocephalus is far more common than most doctors believe. (A large proportion of doctors, including a surprising number of neurologists and psychiatrists are quite unfamiliar with the disorder.)

First, a study in Japan showed that normal pressure hydrocephalus affects a far higher number of individuals than is historically considered possible. Since there are no genetic or racial variations in the incidence of the disease, the figures can be applied globally.

The Japanese researchers investigated 567 individuals aged 65 and older and found seven patients with idiopathic normal pressure hydrocephalus. The researchers conclude 'the prevalence of possible idiopathic normal pressure hydrocephalus to be 1.4%' among individuals aged 65 and older.

When researchers in Sweden investigated the prevalence of probable idiopathic normal pressure hydrocephalus in a population of 65 years and older, they found the incidence to be 4%, with a higher proportion of men than women being diagnosed with the disease.

In the UK, there are approximately 10 million people aged 65 or older. If we use the Japanese figures for the UK's population then it would seem that there are currently around 140,000 people in the UK with normal pressure hydrocephalus. In the US, where there are considerably more than 40 million people aged 65 or older, the Japanese figures would suggest that there are around 560,000 people suffering from normal pressure hydrocephalus. If we use the Swedish figures then it suggests that there are currently 400,000 people in the UK with idiopathic normal pressure hydrocephalus. And in the US the figure is a staggering 1,600,000.

(See the paper entitled 'Prevalence of possible idiopathic normal pressure hydrocephalus in Japan', written by Tanaka, Yamaguchi, Ishikawa, Ishii and Meguro and published by Neuroepidemiology in 2009, and the paper entitled 'Fluid Barriers CNS. Abstracts from Hydrocephalus 2015', written by Rosell CM, Andersson J, Kockum K, Lilija-Lund O, Soderstrom L and Laurell K in Sweden. There are more references about normal pressure hydrocephalus in my short book on the disease entitled *Millions of Alzheimer's Patients Have Been Misdiagnosed (And Could Be Cured)*.)

The research has shown that only a very tiny percentage of these individuals have been accurately diagnosed as suffering from idiopathic normal pressure hydrocephalus. The vast majority of these individuals who have been diagnosed at all will have been diagnosed as suffering from Alzheimer's disease or some other form of dementia or from Parkinson's disease. Many individuals, of course, will not have been given a diagnosis at all but will have been simply labelled 'old' and dismissed as not worthy of attention.

A second way of measuring the incidence of normal pressure hydrocephalus is to look at the incidence of the disease among long-stay patients. The incidence of idiopathic normal pressure hydrocephalus is said to be around 14% among long-term patients in care homes, nursing homes and other residential centres – whether or not they have dementia. This figure suggests that in a small general nursing home with 20 patients, there are likely to be three to six patients who have idiopathic normal pressure hydrocephalus who could be treated and, possibly, cured. In a larger institution, specialising in the care of patients with Alzheimer's disease or some other form of dementia, the figure is likely to be much greater.

A third way of measuring the incidence of normal pressure hydrocephalus is to look at the number of people suffering from dementia in general and then look at studies where attempts have been made to assess the number of patients who have been misdiagnosed.

It is now generally agreed among experts that one in eight individuals over the age of 65 will have Alzheimer's disease. And it is also agreed that patients officially diagnosed as suffering from Alzheimer's disease make up between 50% to 70% of all those suffering from dementia. So the number of people over the age of 65 who have dementia will be between one in four and one in six.

The big question here is: 'How many of the patients diagnosed as suffering from irreversible, untreatable dementia are actually suffering from a disease (idiopathic normal pressure hydrocephalus) for which a cure is available?'

The Hydrocephalus Association in the United States estimates that there are 700,000 adults in America who have idiopathic normal pressure hydrocephalus but that only a fifth of these patients have been diagnosed. The remainder have been misdiagnosed as suffering from Alzheimer's, some other dementia or

Parkinson's disease. Available scientific evidence suggests that the majority of the rest could be treated and restored to good health.

If the Hydrocephalus Association in America is correct, there are 560,000 patients in the US who have idiopathic normal pressure hydrocephalus but who do not know it, have not been diagnosed or treated and who are being left to die, untreated and without hope. The figures for the UK and other countries are undoubtedly similar. The evidence suggests that there are 175,000 patients in the UK who have treatable idiopathic normal pressure hydrocephalus but who have been misdiagnosed as suffering from an untreatable dementia and (since doctors receive a fee for diagnosing it) probably labelled as suffering from Alzheimer's disease.

Around the world there are probably several million patients who have normal pressure hydrocephalus and who could, have been cured if they had been correctly diagnosed.

The key thing to remember is that normal pressure hydrocephalus can be cured with a single, relatively simple surgical procedure. And the bottom line is that patients with dementia, who are confined to a hospital or nursing home or to bed in their own homes, can become independent again if they are treated.

Very few specialist studies have been done to measure the incidence of idiopathic normal pressure hydrocephalus among patients in 'assisted living facilities' or 'extended care facilities' but the results which exist show that between 9% and 14% of the patients studied had idiopathic normal pressure hydrocephalus.

The tragedy, as I have already explained, is that patients with idiopathic normal pressure hydrocephalus are often mistakenly diagnosed as suffering from other disorders such as Alzheimer's disease, other dementias or Parkinson's disease.

'Many people go undiagnosed and untreated because the symptoms of normal pressure hydrocephalus can mimic Alzheimer's disease, Parkinson's disease and other neurological or spinal disorders that can occur in adults as they age', says Michael Williams, a neurologist and director of the Adult Hydrocephalus Center at the Sandra and Malcolm Berman Brain and Spine Institute at Sinai Hospital of Baltimore in Maryland.

The size of this scandal is difficult to comprehend and as the number of people in their 60s and beyond increases, so the number of people with treatable normal pressure hydrocephalus will increase proportionally.

As I mentioned earlier, normal pressure hydrocephalus was first identified in 1965. No one has any idea how many people have been misdiagnosed since then. Because of ignorance among doctors and nurses, idiopathic normal pressure hydrocephalus is rarely diagnosed and so it is invariably categorised as a 'rare disease'.

But idiopathic normal pressure hydrocephalus is not a rare disease. It is clear that when the disease is looked for, it is common.

Once you know what to look out for, idiopathic normal pressure hydrocephalus is not particularly difficult to diagnose. It should not be 'missed' as often as it is. (My mother's diagnosis was missed by a series of neurologists at the Royal Devon and Exeter Hospital. Her case history is described in an appendix at the back of this book.)

The principle symptoms of idiopathic normal pressure hydrocephalus are: a wide-legged, unsteady gait, a tendency to fall a good deal (commonly falling backwards, incontinence (usually urinary but double incontinence sometimes occurs) and dementia. Other symptoms and signs may include headaches. Patients usually appear slow thinking and have impaired memory. They may lose their inhibitions and behave inappropriately in company – saying or doing things that are completely out of character. Patients have difficulty in starting and carrying out tasks, find it hard to focus and lose motivation. They tend to sleep a good deal.

Because other types of dementia may produce similar symptoms, or symptoms which can be confused with these, or because the dementia may be by far the most dominant symptom that it overwhelms the others, it is dangerous to try to make a diagnosis of idiopathic normal pressure hydrocephalus from the symptoms alone.

As a starting point, most doctors investigating dementia and suspecting idiopathic normal pressure hydrocephalus will perform a scan; either an MRI scan or a CT scan. MRI is painless and takes at least half an hour. MRI uses radio signals and a powerful magnet to create a picture of the brain. It will show if the ventricles are enlarged and will provide information about the surrounding brain tissue. An MRI scan will also evaluate the flow of cerebrospinal fluid. An MRI scan provides more information that is likely to be used in making a diagnosis of idiopathic normal pressure hydrocephalus. A CT scan creates a picture of the brain using X-rays and a special scanner. It is reliable, painless and quicker than an MRI and it will show if the ventricles are enlarged or if there is any obvious blockage.

A scan of the brain may show that there is excess cerebrospinal fluid and that the ventricles within the brain are enlarged. Unfortunately, these findings are not pathognomonic – though they certainly suggest that a diagnosis of idiopathic normal pressure hydrocephalus is possible if not probable.

The most accurate way to make a diagnosis is to do a lumbar puncture (also known as a spinal tap) and to remove some of the excess cerebrospinal fluid from around the spinal cord and the brain. If there is an improvement within three or four days after a lumbar puncture has been done and some fluid removed, then the diagnosis of idiopathic normal pressure hydrocephalus is likely. And there is a real chance that the patient's symptoms can be improved.

It is usually wise to allow cerebrospinal fluid to drain for a few days while evaluating the patient.

If there is a clinical improvement after 30 mls or so of fluid have been removed, then there will probably be a good response if a shunt is put into place.

However, the fact that there is no improvement after some cerebrospinal fluid has been removed does not mean that a diagnosis of idiopathic normal pressure hydrocephalus is impossible. It may still be worth putting in a shunt – especially if other signs and symptoms suggest that it might help. It is worth remembering that idiopathic normal pressure hydrocephalus is one of the few diseases masquerading as dementia (and by far the most common) which can be treated effectively.

When a shunt has been placed in situ, it will probably be necessary to adjust the rate at which fluid is draining out. If too much fluid has been allowed out then the patient may develop a headache. The outflow of cerebrospinal fluid can be adjusted without extra surgery. If a shunt is not draining enough fluid then the first symptoms to reoccur will probably be related to walking. The recurrence of a walking problem may mean that the shunt is not working properly or that it needs to be adjusted so that more fluid drains out. It is important to remember that very little research has been done into idiopathic normal pressure hydrocephalus and, in a sense, every patient is an experiment.

There are other tests which may be done to find out whether a patient has idiopathic normal pressure hydrocephalus.

One is the infusion test in which the outflow of cerebrospinal fluid is measured. This test assesses the degree to which the absorption of CSF back into the bloodstream has been blocked.

Another test is to measure the intracranial pressure. A small pressure monitor is inserted through the skull into the brain or the ventricles to measure the intracranial pressure. Unfortunately, this is not necessarily diagnostic since some patients with idiopathic normal pressure hydrocephalus will not have raised intracranial pressure.

A third test, known as isotopic cisternography involves injecting into a radioactive isotope into the lumbar subarachnoid space through a spinal tap. This test allows the absorption of CSF to be evaluated over several days. This test is not particularly often used because it is complicated, and does not reliably predict whether a patient will respond well to shunt surgery.

If a patient is to be properly diagnosed and treated then, in addition to the GP or primary care physician, advice will be needed from a neurologist and a neurosurgeon. There will be two important decisions to make: is the patient suffering from idiopathic normal pressure hydrocephalus and are they likely to benefit from a shunt operation.

Once diagnosed, idiopathic normal pressure hydrocephalus is remarkably simple to treat. And the treatment, a relatively small operation, usually provides a permanent cure. There is no need for long-term drug therapy. (This, I am afraid, explains why the pharmaceutical industry has generally been instrumental in suppressing the interest of the medical profession in the disease. I make no apology for repeating this allegation.)

The aim of treatment is to get rid of the excess cerebrospinal fluid which has accumulated and which is doing the damage. In order to remove the excess fluid, a small piece of plastic tubing (known as a shunt) is placed in the ventricles of the brain and run under the skin to the abdomen where the fluid drains away and is gradually absorbed. This mechanically simple procedure is known as ventriculoperitoneal shunting.

Alternatively, the tubing can lead from the brain to the right atrium of the heart. This is known as ventriculoatrial shunting.

Whatever type of shunt is used, the opening pressure of the valve can be adjusted in order to avoid side effects created by removing too much or too little fluid. This is usually done with the aid of a small magnet which controls the valve's setting and which can be rotated with the aid of a stronger magnet.

Recently, surgeons have begun to perform lumboperitoneal shunt surgery which, it seems, may prove to be safer. A study reported in 2015 suggested that the lumboperitoneal approach is effective. According to Professor S Chabardes, Head of the Functional Stereotactic Unit at the Department of Neurolsurgery of the Joseph Fourier University, Grenoble, France: 'This shunt might be better accepted and tolerated by the patients.'

This sort of treatment definitely works.

Professor G L Lenzi, from the Department of Neurology of La Sapienza, Rome, has stated that: 'patients who had surgery significantly improved motor and non-motor symptoms compared to the non-surgical patients'.

Whatever type of shunt is used, a good response is usually obtained within a few hours of the procedure being performed, with the patient being able to walk more easily and being less incontinent. There is also often a significant improvement in mental function.

The earlier the diagnosis is made, and the earlier treatment is initiated, the greater the chances that the patient's mental capacities will improve. Some early studies suggested that only patients in the early stages of the disease benefitted but more recent studies have shown that putting in a shunt will result in a noticeable or marked improvement in between 70% and 86% of patients who have quite severe symptoms. On the whole, experts have concluded that more than 80% of those having surgery experience improvement. The age of the patient does not seem to have any effect on the outcome. There can be risks with this type of surgery but if the diagnosis has been made then patients and relatives may well feel that the risks are worth taking. Risks in medicine must always be related to the seriousness of the illness involved. If a patient is going to die then even a risky procedure is worth trying.

Much of the important research into idiopathic normal pressure hydrocephalus has taken place in Sweden, and scientists there have developed a way of measuring cerebrospinal fluid dynamics. Artificial cerebrospinal fluid is added and the resultant resistance is measured. The greater the resistance the more likely it is that the patient will benefit from treatment. The scientists also measure the effects of removing 50 mls of cerebrospinal fluid. If tests show an improvement in the patient's ability to think and to move after the removal of the fluid then good results from surgery are much more likely.

Sometimes, patients who have had a good deal of cerebrospinal fluid removed (because a shunt is over-draining, for example) may develop headaches. When this happens the headache can be minimised by using an adjustable shunt.

The prognosis when idiopathic normal pressure hydrocephalus has been diagnosed and treated is excellent. Once the shunt operation is performed, patients with idiopathic normal pressure hydrocephalus will often make quite remarkable recoveries.

It is well known that the human brain can recover after a stroke (in which the tissue may be starved of oxygen by a blood clot or starved of oxygen and compressed by a bleed) and that it is possible for stroke victims to recover lost mental and physical skills for many months after an incident. Similarly, there is no reason why the brain cannot make a remarkable recovery after the traumas of idiopathic normal pressure hydrocephalus although, of course, progress is likely to be faster and more complete when the diagnosis is made at an early stage and the treatment started early.

Around 80% of patients benefit from the shunt surgery offered as treatment, and it is worth remembering that this figure will probably be higher in patients who have good general health and lower in patients who have poor general health and who are suffering from other problems such as diabetes or high blood pressure. The patient who is exceptionally frail and weak is unlikely to do as well as the patient whose only health problem is the idiopathic normal pressure hydrocephalus for which he is being treated.

According to a paper entitled 'Long-term outcome in 109 adult patients operated on for hydrocephalus', which was written by Tisell M, Hellstrom P, Ahl-Borjesson G, Barrows G, Blomsterwall M, Tullberg M, Wikkelso C. and published in the *British Journal of Neurosurgery* in 2006, 79% of patients who responded to a questionnaire after a medium follow-up time of 4.2 years, reported that they still felt improved and 60% had 'persisting observable improvement of gait, living conditions, bladder function and need of sleep'.

It is clear that the majority of patients with idiopathic normal pressure hydrocephalus who are diagnosed and treated with surgery have a clearly beneficial outcome.

It is worth remembering that patients who have the condition and are not treated will continue to deteriorate and will eventually die.

There are, sadly, some (including many in political positions of authority) who do not believe in providing health care for those who have passed a certain age. However, from a purely financial point of view this is nonsense.

Unless society is preparing to introduce mass euthanasia for all patients suffering from dementia then curing a patient, and enabling them to live practical, profitable and useful lives must be preferable in every conceivable way (including financial) to leaving them to be dependent upon 24 hour nursing care, whether that care is provided professionally or by relatives.

The bottom line, however, is that doctors rarely diagnose idiopathic normal pressure hydrocephalus.

If you have a relative or friends whom you think might be suffering from this disorder then you should spare no effort in pushing doctors to consider the diagnosis and to conduct the necessary tests.

Idiopathic normal pressure hydrocephalus was identified in 1965 but even today there is still very little about the disease in medical journals, and medical textbooks devote very little space to the disease. I have in front of me a large medical book which contains over 2,000 pages of closely printed text. Less than half of one page is devoted to idiopathic normal pressure hydrocephalus. I have seen several major medical textbooks which make no mention at all of the disease.

One major textbook, containing nearly 4,000 pages, also devotes just half of one page to normal pressure hydrocephalus and, after dismissing the disease in such a remarkably cavalier fashion adds that 'this disorder accounts for up to 6% of dementias'. Since there are reckoned to be at least 50 million dementia sufferers in the world that would mean that there are approximately 3 million patients in the world with idiopathic normal pressure hydrocephalus – most of them untreated. And this is a disease which can be cured.

If you have never heard of a disease, or you know very little about it, then you are unlikely to think of it when you see a patient suffering from what appears to be a form of dementia. Sadly, the easy thing to do is to make a diagnosis of Alzheimer's disease and abandon the patient to a life of inevitable, remorseless decline. If normal pressure hydrocephalus is untreated then the path of the disease will match that of Alzheimer's disease and no one, least of all the doctor, will question the doctor's diagnosis.

Doctors who have heard of normal pressure hydrocephalus say that it is a rare disease. The fact is, however, that it isn't so much a rare disease as a rarely diagnosed disease. If doctors aren't aware of it and don't look for it then they will never see it.

An important and revealing study done in in Sweden (where the disorder is better known and understood than in most other countries) showed that the majority of doctors considered themselves to have 'poor knowledge' about the symptoms of normal pressure hydrocephalus.

I would suspect that in the UK and the US, the word 'very' could reasonably be placed before the words 'poor knowledge'. My own experience suggests that a majority of doctors have never heard of the disease and therefore never think of it when making a diagnosis of dementia or Alzheimer's disease.

The failure to diagnose normal pressure hydrocephalus has undoubtedly resulted in millions of patients living out the final years of their lives requiring full-time nursing care. How many countless million years of productive life have been wasted? And how many relatives and friends have suffered unnecessarily as they have watched their loved ones die slowly and with a steadily increasing loss of cerebral function?

The pure financial cost of this failure by the medical profession is impossible to estimate accurately. It is estimated that the cost of dementias to the UK is £26.3 billion a year. The country could save between £1.3 billion and £2.6 billion a year by diagnosing and treating patients with idiopathic normal pressure hydrocephalus.

Finally, it is important to remember that relatively little research has been done into this disease and although we do know that it is far commoner than is generally appreciated, there is a desperate need for more research into the causes of the disease as well as into ways of making a rapid diagnosis and new ways to treat the disorder quickly and efficiently.

It is a scandal that this disease has not been investigated more thoroughly.

It is not possible to estimate the emotional, social and financial cost of Alzheimer's disease and dementia. The heartbreak of watching someone you love lose their mind is difficult to explain. And the social and financial cost of looking after a patient suffering from Alzheimer's disease and dementia is impossible to estimate.

If just 1% of the patients currently languishing in hospitals, nursing homes and private homes could be cured then much heartache and billions of dollars would be saved.

It is no exaggeration to say that many millions of patients who require 24 hour nursing care could be returned to useful, independent, productive and rewarding lives if those patients with idiopathic normal pressure hydrocephalus were correctly diagnosed and not merely dismissed as suffering from an incurable dementia.

Vast amounts of money are spent by medical researchers – sometimes on disorders which affect very few patients.

Vast amounts of publicity are given to disorders which are genuinely rare.

So, why is idiopathic normal pressure hydrocephalus so little known?

And why is so little effort put into researching the disorder?

Part of the answer is that very little money is spent on researching or publicising disorders which affect the elderly. Disorders which affect those over 60 are regarded as unglamorous and therefore not worth the attention of politicians, doctors, nurses or journalists.

But the main answer, I'm afraid, lies in the way that medical research is conducted.

Most medical research is organised and paid for by drug companies looking for new products to sell. Doctors and scientists hoping to be given grants will usually look for a drug solution to any problem because they know that the best way to obtain drug company money is to offer a possibly valuable therapeutic solution to a chronic problem. Similarly, many charities have links with drug companies. And they too will be keen to make it clear that money given to them will be spent on searching for a solution which involves a solution which can be patented and then prescribed or sold over the counter.

There is no need to find a pharmaceutical solution to idiopathic normal pressure hydrocephalus because we already know how to cure the disease. A relatively simple one-off operation will provide a long-term cure. There is no opportunity for a researcher or a charity to offer a drug company a profitable outcome if they help pay for a research programme into the disease.

And so little or no research is done.

And since many of the world's medical journals are effectively controlled by drug companies (which provide the advertising which keeps the journals alive) there are few articles drawing attention to a disease which the medical profession has more or less forgotten.

So idiopathic normal pressure hydrocephalus remains almost unknown.

If you suspect that a relative or friend might have idiopathic normal pressure hydrocephalus then you must take action.

Remember: whenever a diagnosis of Alzheimer's disease or any other type of dementia is made then it is wise to seek a second or third opinion. Similarly, when a diagnosis of Parkinson's disease is made another opinion should be sought. Idiopathic normal pressure hydrocephalus is often missed but it can be treated with spectacular, life-saving results.

'People shouldn't assume that all dementia is incurable Alzheimer's and that their situation is hopeless,' says neurosurgeon Ann Marie Flannery, a member of the joint guidelines committee of the American Association of Neurological Surgeons and Congress of Neurological Surgeons.

Michael Williams, the neurologist, says that 'the literature in the past 15 years shows that if you conduct the right tests and select the right patients, the likelihood of benefit is quite high and the risk of harm is quite low.'

Writing as the relative of a patient who had the disease, and having seen the effects of idiopathic normal pressure hydrocephalus far closer than I would have liked, I would say that the risks of performing the shunting operation are always worth taking if a diagnosis of idiopathic normal pressure hydrocephalus is probable or even possible. When a patient is demented, bed bound and doubly incontinent the potential upside is dramatic and the guaranteed downside is of limited consequence.

And the simple fact is that everyone will benefit if more patients are properly diagnosed. Treating idiopathic normal pressure hydrocephalus in the elderly population will reduce health care expenditure dramatically, making hospital beds available for more acute patients.

It is in all our interests to put more time, energy and money into investigating idiopathic normal pressure hydrocephalus and doing more to educate the public, the medical profession and the nursing profession about a disease which is a surprisingly common cause of dementia and the only common cause of dementia which can be treated and cured.

Chapter Four

Alzheimer's Disease

At any age, few things are more frightening than the idea of losing your mind.

And, as a result of work done by drug companies, doctors, charities and journalists, for most people 'losing your mind' means developing Alzheimer's disease. For an increasing number of people over 50, this nightmare is becoming a reality.

Alzheimer's disease was virtually unheard of just a few decades ago. Today, Alzheimer's disease is described as an epidemic.

Scientists have claimed that Alzheimer's disease is commoner now because people are living longer. This is nonsense. Visit any cemetery and the chances are high that you will find plenty of graves for people who died in their 80s or 90s around 100 years ago. (You will also find plenty of graves for young children – showing just how high the incidence of infant and child mortality used to be and why the average life expectancy was so short.)

The incidence of Alzheimer's disease has risen partly because the size of the population has increased. If there are twice as many people living in a town then the incidence of dementia in the town will probably increase in proportion. And the incidence of Alzheimer's will continue to rise steadily as the population increases.

But the alleged incidence of Alzheimer's disease has also risen because there are strong commercial incentives for this diagnosis to be made erroneously. A diagnosis of Alzheimer's disease should never be made until all other possible causes of dementia have been excluded but, as I have already shown, that is not what happens.

Alzheimer's is, like all forms of dementia, a terrible disease: gradually robbing the sufferer of his or her memory, judgement, reasoning skills, speech and dignity. The disease also has an effect on the emotions as well as on behaviour.

Here are three basic facts:

Alzheimer's, a physical, progressive condition for which there is no known cure, causes degeneration of the nerve cells in the cerebral cortex of the brain as well as loss of brain mass.

Alzheimer's affects both men and women; no sex or nationality is immune to the disease.

The incidence of Alzheimer's seems to increases with age: it occurs in up to 30 per cent of people over the age of 85. However, although this is uncommon,

Alzheimer's disease can affect people as young as 35. When it occurs at an early age, Alzheimer's is known as early-onset familial Alzheimer's disease and it tends to progress much more rapidly than late-onset Alzheimer's. For many years, early-onset Alzheimer's was known as pre-senile dementia (dementia that is not associated with advanced age). Early-onset Alzheimer's disease can be an inherited disease. It is important to repeat, by the way, that there is no reason why mental faculties should deteriorate with age. Dementia is not a normal consequence of growing old.

Dementia (which is a Latin word meaning 'loss of mind') is a gradual deterioration in mental function: affecting memory, thinking, judgement, concentration, learning, speech and behaviour. Because the disease begins very gradually, the symptoms of Alzheimer's may go unnoticed for a while.

Mild forgetfulness, which is so common in the early stages of the disease, may simply be put down to 'getting older' (though it is worth repeating that there is no specific reason why memory should deteriorate with age).

However, as the disease progresses, the symptoms become more noticeable, especially the memory loss. It is usually the loss of memory that motivates sufferers or their relatives to seek medical attention.

Not every sufferer of Alzheimer's will follow the course of the disease exactly. The disease, which usually develops gradually, progresses faster in some people than it does in others.

It is also important to be aware that even though the commonest symptoms of the disease are shared by the majority of sufferers, no two people will experience identical symptoms.

The symptoms which appear on the list below are not inevitable. But knowing a little about the possible progression of Alzheimer's can help you plan for the future. Forewarned is forearmed.

The following symptoms usually occur in the early stages of Alzheimer's disease:

Forgetfulness, especially of recent events. Sufferers may remember events that took place a year ago, but lose all recollection of what occurred an hour ago. In the very early stages of Alzheimer's, it is only short-term memory loss which is affected; memory loss deteriorates as the disease progresses. It is not uncommon for sufferers to become highly defensive when questioned about their failing memory; this is because they usually feel embarrassed or frightened by it. Some sufferers even go to great lengths to hide their memory loss from friends and relatives.

Difficulty in making decisions.

An inability to do tasks which require some intellectual ability, such as simple mathematical calculations, managing the household finances, etc.

Repetitious questioning – the same question may be asked over and over again because the sufferer has lost all memory of having asked that question previously. Stories may also be repeated for the same reason.

Misplacing objects – the sugar may be put in the fridge for example, because the sufferer is not able to remember where it is normally stored.

Constantly losing things.

Difficulty in finding the right word when talking (Anomia).

Frequently losing train of thought during conversations.

Apathy.

Forgetting the names of objects and calling them by a different name, for example, a chair may be called a bench or a cupboard might be called a wardrobe.

Loss of concentration.

Forgetting familiar names.

Listlessness.

Inability to learn new information – this is due to loss of short-term memory which is essential when it comes to learning anything new.

Depression and anxiety.

Sleep disturbances.

Disorientation in time – a sufferer may be confused as to what day, month or year it is.

Poor judgement – the Alzheimer sufferer may put on a thick woolly jumper even though it's the middle of summer and the temperature is ninety degrees in the shade.

Increasing difficulty with speech. The sufferer may withdraw from intellectual conversations as a result.

Personality changes – a previously trusting person may suddenly become suspicious of everyone they encounter, even their loved ones. Other personality changes may include: hostility, jealousy, outbursts of anger and sometimes violence.

Getting lost in familiar places. So, for example, a sufferer may forget their usual route back home from a shop or from a friend's house.

Symptoms usually occurring in the later stages of Alzheimer's disease include:

Carelessness – frequently leaving the cooker on or, if they smoke, leaving burning cigarettes lying around. This type of carelessness can be life-threatening both to the sufferer as well as to the people around them.

Mood swings – sobbing uncontrollably one minute and laughing hysterically the next for no apparent reason.

Simple everyday tasks becoming increasingly difficult.

Lack of personal hygiene.

Personality changes becoming more apparent.

Increasing problems with speech.

Wandering – roaming from room to room as if looking for something.

Repetition of simple but usually purposeful activities. For instance, repeatedly smoothing down a fold in the tablecloth.

Behaviour may become increasingly bizarre.

Severe deterioration of comprehension.

Loss of sexual inhibitions.

Strong denial that anything is wrong.

Extreme lack of motivation.

Severe sleep disturbances.

Symptoms usually occurring in the advanced stages of Alzheimer's disease include:

A failure to recognize familiar faces. The patient may not be able to identify their spouse and may confuse him/her with another family member. It is also quite common for sufferers not even to recognize themselves when they look in the mirror and because of this, they may complain of a stranger being in the room.

The sufferer can no longer find his or her way around their own home.

Loss of the ability to read and write.

Personality changes becoming more severe and problematical.

The sufferer may experience hallucinations.

A complete failure to recognize ordinary, everyday objects.

Speech becomes unintelligible.

A total dependency on others for help with: toileting, bathing, eating, dressing, etc.

Bowel and bladder incontinence.

An inability to walk or even sit up.

Severe confusion and disorientation.

Paranoid delusions.

An inability to swallow.

Finally, there is likely to be a complete loss of memory and speech as well as muscle function. A patient with final stage Alzheimer's disease will need complete nursing care for they will be unable to do anything for themselves.

Death usually occurs in about five to ten years after diagnosis (always dying of something else since Alzheimer's disease itself does not cause death – see Appendix at the back of this book) though in some cases, the sufferer can have the disease for as long as 20 years.

Sufferers do not die from the primary brain damage caused by Alzheimer's, but from a complication of the disease. This is a consequence of the increasing debility that the disease causes to the sufferer. Once sufferers become immobile, they are far more susceptible to infection and to the development of heart disease.

Finally, it is important to point out that individuals who experience some or all of the symptoms associated with Alzheimer's should not panic. Most of us experience lapses of memory from time to time during conversation. These lapses of memory are quite normal.

However, if forgetfulness becomes noticeably worse, it is time to seek help. Remember that the symptoms of Alzheimer's can be caused by a wide variety of illnesses, some of which can be treated. If a doctor assumes that dementia is caused by Alzheimer's then it would probably be wise to find another doctor.

Making a firm diagnosis of Alzheimer's is not easy. To be 100 per cent certain that someone is suffering from Alzheimer's disease, an autopsy on the brain needs to be performed. The next best option is for a specialist to carry out some tests to try to make an accurate diagnosis. The tests, which are performed to help diagnose Alzheimer's disease, are sometimes said to be about 90 per cent accurate although I have grave doubts about this. Plaques on the brain can occur with Alzheimer's but they can nearly always be seen on an older brain and so their significance is probably overstated. With the aid of state-of-the-art equipment, researchers claim they are becoming increasingly adept at spotting the disease but the diagnosis is really one that should only be made when all other possibilities have been excluded.

When doctors suspect that a patient might have Alzheimer's disease, they should perform the following tests:

Psychiatric examination – this is to rule out depression or any other mental illness that can mimic the symptoms of Alzheimer's disease.

Blood tests – to detect illnesses (such as vitamin B12 deficiency) that can cause dementia-type symptoms.

Mental test – to assess brain function such as: memory, the ability to do simple addition or subtraction, comprehension, etc.

EMG (Electromyography) – to test the large muscles in the body. (In some diseases of the brain, this activity can malfunction.)

Neurological examination – the nervous system is examined to look for other illnesses which might be causing similar symptoms, such as Parkinson's disease, previous strokes, brain tumours, etc.

CAT scan (Computerised Axial Tomography) – takes pictures of the brain to check for any anomalies.

Physical examination – like the neurological and the blood tests, this examination is also used to rule out any other underlying disorders.

EEG (Electroencephalogram) – to assess abnormalities in brain wave activity.

Medical history assessment – this may involve interviews with the patient and his or her partner or with one or two members of his/her family. This is to find out how he/she is functioning with day-to-day living and to learn about any previous or any familial illnesses. It is also important to assess drug therapy to see if prescription drug use could be causing confusion and memory loss.

MRI scan (Magnetic Resonance Imaging) – is very much like the CAT scan. An MRI scan may be used if nothing shows up from the CAT scan.

SPECT scan (Single Photon Emission Computerised Tomography) – unlike the MRI and the CAT scanners which look at the structure of the brain, the SPECT scan looks for a change in the function of brain tissue. The person being scanned is given an injection of glucose together with a mild radioactive material. This substance, called radionuclide, circulates in the brain. The SPECT scan then measures the amount of radionuclide in various parts of brain tissue. (The brain's main source of energy is glucose; in people suffering with Alzheimer's, certain areas of the brain do not absorb as much glucose as would be normal.)

If there is any suspicion that the symptoms of dementia could be caused by normal pressure hydrocephalus then a lumbar puncture should be performed.

Sadly, most diagnoses of dementia (and, by default, of Alzheimer's disease) are made without most (or any) of these tests being performed. That is, in my view, criminal negligence.

Although it is important to get a diagnosis as early on in the disease as possible, because this enables everyone concerned to plan for the future, it is also a good idea to retain an open mind. It is by no means uncommon for new symptoms or signs to appear and for these to suggest that an alternative diagnosis is the correct one.

It is, incidentally, important to remember that most doctors still dramatically under-estimate the importance of iatrogenesis – or doctor-induced disease. It is perfectly possible for a team of doctors to perform all these tests and yet forget to find out if a patient is taking a tranquilliser or sedative which could be causing all the symptoms. And even when the doctors know that a patient is taking prescription drugs they are likely to ignore, forget or downplay the possible side effects of prescription drug therapy.

Appendices

Appendix One

Case History: Antoinette Coleman

For some time Antoinette, my wife, had suffered from painful muscle spasms, sensory loss, memory loss and a whole host of other symptoms. In 2005, a blood test showed a vitamin B12 level of 264. At the time, this was regarded as within normal levels and doctors looked elsewhere for a cause of her symptoms. We now know that this level of Vitamin B12 should have set alarm bells ringing.

In 2009, Antoinette was referred to a specialist neurologist who then referred her onwards to Dr Peter Heywood at Frenchay Hospital in Bristol. Unfortunately, Dr Heywood was not available for the appointment and so Antoinette saw a fairly young registrar called Dr Coulthard.

Dr Coulthard thought Antoinette might have a tumour on her spine and ordered an urgent MRI scan of Antoinette's brain and spine. Ten days later, we went back to the hospital for the MRI scan. Once again Dr Peter Heywood, the consultant, wasn't available and Antoinette saw the same registrar as before. The scan showed no signs of any tumour. However, when the registrar examined Antoinette, she found brisk reflexes, fasciculation in her tongue, upgoing plantars and muscle weakness. This time the doctor decided that Antoinette might be suffering from motor neurone disease.

We visited the hospital a total of four times. Multiple sclerosis was thought of and considered as a diagnosis. We never saw the consultant to whom Antoinette had been referred. Maybe Dr Peter Heywood had retired or left and the system has not yet registered that he has disappeared. Maybe he was just too busy.

In the end, we had to telephone the hospital several times to find out if Antoinette had motor neurone disease. Eventually, we discovered that the registrar was off sick and that the letter telling Antoinette the diagnosis had been typed and was sitting waiting to be signed. A secretary said that the letter would be sent when ready. I then pointed out that we have been waiting nearly three weeks to find out whether or not Antoinette had a fatal disease. Eventually, after some pressure, the hospital confirmed that Antoinette did not have motor neurone disease. Antoinette sensibly decided that she'd had enough of Frenchay Hospital. She didn't return.

We now jump forwards ten years.

In April 2019, Antoinette decided that the tiredness from which she was suffering was becoming unbearable. Her other symptoms were also getting steadily worse and she was regularly visiting the terrifying outskirts of dementia at just 46-years-old. She was losing her memory and was severely depressed and tearful.

Since the specialists at Frenchay had investigated multiple sclerosis and motor neurone disease and since both those diseases can progress at unpredictable speeds, it seemed apparent that Antoinette's condition (whichever it was) was merely progressing at its own speed. However, it did not seem unlikely that there might be something else (such as simple anaemia) contributing to the tiredness which Antoinette felt.

By this time, Antoinette's symptoms had become intolerable (and remarkably akin to those associated with multiple sclerosis).

Here is a list of her symptoms which she prepared for her doctor:

Tinnitus
Tingling, stinging and burning pains
Partial numbness
Muscle spasms
A tendency to trip up
Vision problems
Memory problems
Auditory hallucinations
Tiredness
Brain fog
Dizziness
Anxiety
Depression
Suicidal thoughts
Irritability to loud noises
Weakness in the legs
Impaired sense of smell and taste
Palpitations
Poor balance
Sleep disturbance
Bladder problems

Those are all symptoms which occur with vitamin B12 deficiency. In Antoinette's case, this was definitely not a dietary problem but almost certainly an absorption problem.

Fortunately, her GP did a vitamin B12 test.

This was our first lucky break.

The second lucky break was that Antoinette's serum vitamin B12 level was just below the absurdly low figure used by the local laboratory as an acceptable low level. If her vitamin B12 had been just a little higher, the diagnosis would have been missed. Again.

As I write this (May 2019) Antoinette has just completed her first course of vitamin B12 injections. There are already some signs of improvement. She will now start the long, slow process of recovery.

If she hadn't visited the GP, and had that blood test, she would have continued to deteriorate.

There is no doubt in my mind that the specialist neurologists who saw Antoinette should have made the correct diagnosis over a decade ago. The diagnosis was missed because her vitamin B12 level was erroneously considered to be normal.

Appendix Two

Facts about vitamin B12 deficiency

Vitamin B12 is essential for the formation of red blood cells but also for a good deal else. If your body is short of vitamin B12 you are likely to develop a form of anaemia known as pernicious anaemia. The size of your individual red blood cells will be increased but their number will be reduced. The word pernicious was originally added to the diagnosis because the disorder always ended in death.

Vitamin B12 also plays a vital part in the working of the central nervous system, and a long-term shortage of the vitamin can lead to damage being done to the brain and spinal cord. Vitamin B12 aids the production of genetic matter inside cells which is needed for the creation of new cells.

Vitamin B12 is an unusual vitamin in that before it can be absorbed into the body it needs to be linked to a substance called 'intrinsic factor' which is formed in the stomach. There are a number of reasons why 'intrinsic factor' may be missing. Patients who have had stomach surgery may be unable to produce this 'intrinsic factor'. This problem is less common these days now that ulcer healing drugs have made many stomach operations obsolete.

Vegans, and sometimes vegetarians, may also find themselves short of vitamin B12 because their diet doesn't contain enough vitamin B12 rich foods. And those with inflammatory bowel disorders are likely to become deficient in vitamin B12. Indeed, it is so easy to become short of this vitamin, that around 20% of all those over 60 years of age are likely to be short of vitamin B12. That makes vitamin B12 deficiency one of the commonest serious disorders known to man.

Vitamin B12 is found in many animal products — including meat, eggs and dairy produce. It is also available in tempeh, soya milk, edible seaweeds, dried spirulina and a wide range of fortified products now available (including cereals, margarines, textured vegetable proteins and fortified yeast extracts and savoury spreads). Vitamin B12 is manufactured by micro-organisms such as yeasts, bacteria, moulds and some algae. Vitamin B12 is also found in beer, cider, fermented soya foods (such as soy sauce), barley malt syrup and parsley. The most reliable vegan sources of B12 are foods fortified with the vitamin. Soya products (such as soya milks), breakfast cereals, yeast extracts and margarines are particularly likely to contain added vitamin B12.

Vegan women who are pregnant and vegan mothers who intend to breast feed their babies should make sure that they eat foods which are fortified with vitamin B12.

The human body can store this vitamin for long periods (up to five or six years), so a daily dietary source is not necessary. In addition, the healthy body recycles this vitamin very effectively, recovering it from bile and other intestinal secretions, which is why the dietary requirement is so low.

Appendix Three

Signs and Symptoms caused by low vitamin B12

Of all the vitamins, the one known as vitamin B12 seems to be the one which can cause the widest variety of troublesome signs and symptoms in the human body.

A deficiency of vitamin B12 can affect the body in many ways. It can:

Damage blood cell production: with symptoms including anaemia, tiredness, weakness, enlarged spleen and enlarged liver.

Damage the central nervous system, causing widespread demyelination and affecting the brain: the symptoms can include unsteadiness, numbness, tingling, burning, muscle weakness, paralysis, balance problems, difficulty in walking, depression, visual disturbances, incontinence, memory loss, disturbances in taste and smell, shaking, cramps, abnormal reflexes, confusion and dementia.

Damage the immune system causing an increased susceptibility to infection, poor wound healing and an exaggerated and potentially dangerous response to vaccinations.

Damage the musculo-skeletal system causing osteoporosis and bone fractures.

Damage the vascular system producing heart symptoms (such as palpitations and tachycardia), breathlessness (particularly on exercise) chest pain and the symptoms of congestive heart failure.

Damage the gastrointestinal tract producing indigestion, malabsorption, constipation, weight loss and abdominal pains.

Damage the genitourinary tract producing impotence, infertility and cystitis and complicating surgical procedures.

It should be clear from this list that Vitamin B12 deficiency can mimic a wide range or disorders – and lead to inaccurate diagnoses.

I have already explained, earlier in this book, that vitamin B12 deficiency can lead to dementia and be mistaken for Alzheimer's disease. Since Alzheimer's disease is progressive and incurable, such a mistake can be disastrous. I have no doubt that many patients still incarcerated in institutions, could be partially or completely cured if they were tested for vitamin B12 deficiency, properly diagnosed and treated effectively with a few cheap injections of vitamin B12.

There are, however, many other diseases which can also be diagnosed by mistake when the patient really has an easily treatable vitamin B12 deficiency.

Multiple sclerosis is probably the most obvious disorder in this category (and I have no doubt that thousands of patients whose lives have been devastated by a wrong diagnosis of this disorder could now be living perfectly normal lives). Patients with vitamin B12 deficiency are commonly diagnosed with tumours, motor neurone disease, circulatory disease, mental disease and many more.

The misdiagnosing of patients who have nothing more complicated than simple vitamin B12 deficiency is without doubt the most egregious example of iatrogenesis I have come across in a lifetime assessing doctor-induced disease. Vitamin B12 deficiency is an epidemic and I have no doubt that a simple blood test, properly assessed, would lead to the re-evaluation of millions of mistaken diagnoses.

Appendix Four

Case histories: patients with normal pressure hydrocephalus

(Versions of these case histories previously appeared in my book about NPH which is entitled *Millions of Alzheimer's Patients Have Been Misdiagnosed (And Could Be Cured)*.)

1. Professor Emeritus of Hepatology Harold O Conn MD FACP of the Yale University School of Medicine in the US, developed problems with walking shortly after retiring. He was 68-years-old when the symptoms started. They gradually became more pronounced. Dr Conn was diagnosed by colleagues in the department of neurology at Yale University as suffering from 'Parkinson's disease like syndrome. Dr Conn's wife noticed that her husband was losing his sense of humour and his ability to concentrate. He also developed double incontinence. Three more eminent neurologists were consulted and they diagnosed a variant of Parkinson's Disease. Their prognosis was poor. At a follow up appointment five years after they made their diagnosis, they predicted that the cerebral atrophy would continue and that the professor's symptoms would get worse. They also said that the condition was untreatable. Nine years after the initial symptoms had appeared, when he was 77-years-old, Dr Conn could barely walk. He was then seen by a neurologist in another state. The new neurologist made a diagnosis of idiopathic normal pressure hydrocephalus. When 60 mls of cerebrospinal fluid was removed, Dr Conn made an immediate improvement. And after shunt surgery was performed, Dr Conn improved permanently. He had had the disease for 10 years and had repeatedly been wrongly diagnosed by specialists working in one of the world's premier medical schools.

2. A 40-year-old widow and housewife, Mrs LCB was referred from the General Outpatient Department of the Jos University Teaching Hospital to the hospital's psychiatric unit in May 2014. She had eight weeks history of recurrent vomiting, recurrent headaches, fearfulness and withdrawal. She had been in good health up until the start of that period of illness. The patient's headache was described as generalised, throbbing and non-radiating and it was mildly relieved with analgesics. There was some dizziness and blurring of vision. She had some fever, felt weak and could walk only with support. Since the patient had recently witnessed gunshots in Nigeria, an initial diagnosis of Post-Traumatic Stress Disorder was made. Two weeks after admission to the psychiatric unit, the patient had a convulsion and also complained of

progressive weakness of her lower limbs and of urinary incontinence both during the day and at night. Her speech also became irrational and she had visual hallucinations. At that point, a diagnosis of Generalised Tonic Clonic seizure was made. A CT scan revealed idiopathic normal pressure hydrocephalus. The patient had a ventriculo-peritoneal shunt surgery. Following the surgery, the patient did well and all symptoms subsided. The patient was able to walk with minimal support. The doctors looking after this patient reported that in their experience, idiopathic normal pressure hydrocephalus can be relieved successfully with a shunt implanted surgically to drain excess cerebrospinal fluid. The details of this patient were reported in the *Journal of Neurological Disorders*. The article was entitled 'Normal Pressure Hydrocephalus with Onset Following a Traumatic Experience'. The author of the article was Aishatu Yusha'u Armiya'u of the Department of Psychiatry, Jos University Teaching Hospital, Jos, Plateau State, Nigeria.

3. Bob Fowler was so convinced that he was dying that he wrote his own obituary. He had, in his own words, 'been to doctor after doctor after doctor with absolutely no positive results'. For nine years, Mr Fowler increasingly suffered with trouble walking, memory problems and difficulty controlling his urination. Eventually, Mr Fowler developed severe dementia, had to stop working and was confined to a wheelchair. After some years, his wife began making plans to put him a nursing home. Finally, Mr Fowler met a doctor who recognised that he had idiopathic normal pressure hydrocephalus. After surgery, Mr Fowler literally got up out of his wheelchair and resumed his life. The change was dramatic. 'All of a sudden I felt fantastic,' he said. 'I'm 74-years-old now, and I'm doing things I wouldn't have dreamed of doing anytime during my 60s.' Mr Fowler went back to work, started playing golf, driving his car and spending time with his family. This case history was discovered on the internet.

4. Retired dentist Milton Newman suffered for 15 years with loss of memory and concentration. Mr Newman's symptoms started when he was about 55-years-old. 'Reading a book was difficult because I couldn't remember what happened 10 pages back. And later on, conversation was difficult because I'd forget what people would say.' Eventually Mr Newman was diagnosed as suffering from Alzheimer's disease. He regarded the diagnosis as a death sentence. Finally, after years of suffering, Mr Newman, met a doctor who diagnosed idiopathic normal pressure hydrocephalus. Surgery reduced the symptoms immediately. 'I felt like the old Milton,' said Mr Newman. This case history was discovered on the internet.

5. A 70-year-old woman suffered a gradual onset of gait disturbance and later on developed dementia and occasional urinary incontinence. For two years, her mental problems got worse and her ability to walk deteriorated to the point where she was unable to walk and care for herself at home. She became a

hospital patient in Norway after she had first noticed her symptoms. A CT scan showed ventricular enlargement out of proportion to the cerebral atrophy. When a lumbar puncture was performed, it was found that the CSF pressure was raised. When a shunt operation was performed, the patient gradually improved and a year later she was able to live normally at home. Her dementia had improved considerably, her urinary incontinence had disappeared and her gait was almost normal. This case history was discovered on the internet.

6. This is a rather long case history and it was painful to write because it describes the final year of my mother's life.

I have no doubt that if the incompetent staff at two hospitals in Devon had been a little more alert, and a little less arrogant, my mother could have been cured. She had idiopathic normal pressure hydrocephalus but, despite her obvious symptoms, and much prompting, the diagnosis was ignored.

My wife (who has no formal medical training) initially made the correct diagnosis by keying my mother's symptoms and signs into a search engine. We agreed that idiopathic normal pressure hydrocephalus was by far the most likely diagnosis. Although I qualified as a GP, the disease was not one with which I was well acquainted. The disease fitted my mother's symptoms perfectly. She had an unusual wide-legged walk. She had a tendency to fall. And she had urinary incontinence. She was also showing signs of dementia. These are precisely the symptoms shown by patients with idiopathic normal pressure hydrocephalus.

We repeatedly suggested the diagnosis of idiopathic normal pressure hydrocephalus but specialist after specialist rejected it until it was too late. They seemed bizarrely desperate to settle on every possible diagnosis that wasn't the right one and in retrospect I can only believe it was because they too knew little or nothing about idiopathic normal pressure hydrocephalus.

I also fear that she was treated superficially because of her age (she was 83 when her symptoms started but had been in excellent health). Today, everyone needs to be aware that patients over the age of 70 are regularly regarded as second class citizens by doctors, nurses and other hospital staff. Sadly, I do not think that this attitude is uncommon. Medical staff take little interest in patients who are over 70 years of age, and this lack of concern has been endorsed and encouraged by politicians. The United Nations has introduced Sustainable Development Goals which allow governments and health services to discriminate against anyone over the age of 70 on the grounds that people who die when they are over 70-years-old cannot be said to have died prematurely, and so will not count when a nation's healthcare is being assessed. The Sustainable Development Goals give politicians the authority to ignore the health needs of citizens who have reached their 'three score years and ten' and who are regarded by society's accountants as an economic burden. Indeed, there is, a regrettably widespread assumption in hospitals everywhere that anyone who is over 70 must simply learn to live with their problems and adapt to changes which are simply an inevitable part of the ageing process. The Liverpool Care Pathway, which entitles doctors and nurses to withhold food, water and essential treatment from patients who are over the age of 65 and who are, therefore, regarded as an expensive nuisance is still used as a guideline by many doctors and nurses and hospital bureaucrats who are searching for ways to clear 'blocked beds' and reduce nursing costs.

During my mother's illness, I repeatedly contacted her GP in Budleigh Salterton and I spoke and wrote regularly to the vast variety of doctors at the hospital in Exeter – frequently suggesting that my mother was suffering from normal pressure hydrocephalus. However, the doctors and nurses seemed concerned only to produce diagnoses which were untreatable and terminal. Only at the end, when it was too late to do anything, did they agree that she had all along been suffering from idiopathic normal pressure hydrocephalus.

My mother's story begins when, in October 2004, she first had difficulty in walking. She was mentally alert. Suddenly, in November 2004, after a rapid deterioration, it was decided that she was suffering from terminal cancer with metastases. She was not considered healthy enough for palliative radiotherapy and was described, by her consultant oncologist, as 'frail, confused, bedbound and dependent'. She had to be catheterised because she was incontinent. The idea of rehabilitation was abandoned because of her alleged terminal cancer. A neurologist who assessed her mental state reported that my mother did not know where she was and had failed to recognise the doctor. She was given the usual simple mental test (date of birth and so on) and scored 0 out of 10. My father was telephoned at home and told that my mother was terminally ill with cancer and that there were metastatic deposits in her spine, lung and possibly liver. It was thought that her mental condition could be caused by secondaries in her brain. No one knew what sort of cancer she was suffering from or where the primary was situated.

A cancer specialist told me that my mother either had cancer of the breast or the lung with secondaries and was too weak for treatment. 'That's the nature of the beast', she said. She told me that there was no hope. She turned out to be completely wrong in everything other than the fact that there was no hope.

On Sunday 21st November 2004, we noticed that my mother's urine bag was red. There was clearly blood in her urine. A nurse had changed the catheter bag several times without bothering to report to anyone that the urine in the bag was red with blood. Or perhaps they hadn't noticed. I reported the blood and a doctor put my mother on amoxicillin for a urinary infection. After the blood appeared in the urine, the cancer specialist told me that my mother had secondaries in her kidneys. By the 30th November, the urine was clear and the bag was no longer red. The diagnosis of cancer secondaries in the kidneys was never withdrawn, though it too was completely wrong.

My mother stayed in the Exeter hospital, which is a teaching hospital, for the next few months. Numerous consultants saw her and decided that there was nothing to be done. Just about every different doctor came up with their own favourite diagnosis but although my wife and I repeatedly suggested that my mother might be suffering from idiopathic normal pressure hydrocephalus, no one seemed keen to accept this solution. My mother's symptoms now seemed to defy diagnosis. She managed to get out of bed occasionally but was unsteady on her feet. And she had developed a rather strange way of walking with her feet wide apart.

Idiopathic normal pressure hydrocephalus is not something GPs see very much at all. But it is the sort of thing teaching hospital neurologists really should know about. I had never seen a patient with it. The doctors looking after my mother dismissed the diagnosis of idiopathic normal pressure hydrocephalus and stuck with their neoplastic madness. There was never a shred of evidence in support of that diagnosis.

The care my mother received was appalling. She spent virtually all her time in bed, becoming steadily weaker. We couldn't move my mother to a private hospital because she has not yet been diagnosed and clearly a private hospital would not have the investigative wherewithal. When I asked if I could send in private physiotherapists, I was told that I could not. The nurses on the ward did not seem to have heard of the danger of deep vein thrombosis or the need to avoid pressure sores by moving patients around. On occasion, my mother would also throw off all her clothes and we would have to rush to draw the screens while we fought to pull the bed covers over her. The nurses didn't come because the ward had been designed in such a way that from the nurses' station it was difficult if not impossible for nurses to see what was happening on the ward. Once, I sat beside my mother's bed when two nurses arrived. One said: 'Have you had a drink this morning?' 'Yes thank you,' said my mother, who had been officially declared demented and mentally incompetent. 'Right.' said the nurse. She wrote this information down on the fluids chart she was carrying. The cold cup of tea was standing, untouched, on the bed table in front of my mother. If we hadn't helped her to drink, I firmly believe that my mother would have died of dehydration. Maybe that was the idea.

At one point during her stay in the Exeter hospital, my mother had a diagnostic lumbar puncture and a quantity of cerebrospinal fluid was removed. Immediately afterwards, she improved noticeably. For a day or two she seemed stronger and her mental function began to improve. It seemed to me that the improvement was significant and suggested that there had been too much fluid around my mother's brain. It seemed likely that the lumbar puncture, by removing some of the fluid, had reduced the pressure and alleviated her symptoms.

The doctors to whom I mentioned this, dismissed my suggestion and insisted that the improvement was simply a coincidence. What would a former GP and writer of books know about these things? No one actually patted me on the head but it felt as though they had done so.

After my mother had finally been diagnosed as suffering from idiopathic normal pressure hydrocephalus (just before she died) I managed to find this in a large medical textbook: 'To help with the diagnosis, doctors do a spinal tap (lumbar puncture) to remove excess cerebrospinal fluid. If this procedure relieves symptoms, idiopathic normal pressure hydrocephalus is likely, and treatment is likely to be effective.' There are very few devastating diseases that can be cured so cheaply, so quickly and so permanently.

On Monday 25th April 2005, the neurology registrar at the Royal Devon and Exeter hospital announced that my mother's prognosis was bleak although they still hadn't made a diagnosis. The cancer diagnosis had now been abandoned. I was told that six neurologists and numerous other consultants had seen her and that every conceivable test had been done. The registrar told me that it would be difficult to find a nursing home capable of looking after her. In addition to her physical paralysis, she was again diagnosed as suffering from dementia. I was told that this could be vascular or a consequence of possible encephalitis. It seemed clear that my mother needed to stay in hospital for the rest of her life.

On Tuesday 26th April 2005, my mother was, at my request, moved to Budleigh hospital so that my father, who lived in Budleigh Salterton, could visit more easily. For six months he had visited the Exeter hospital once or twice a day to feed my mother (who would otherwise have almost certainly starved to death). I also wanted my mother out of the hospital in Exeter because I wasn't terribly impressed by the nursing care she had received. If I had to choose two words to describe the hospital care, they would be 'apathetic' and 'neglectful'.

The hospital in Budleigh was clearly what used to be a cottage hospital – suitable for providing nursing care for local patients.

On Wednesday 27th April 2005, at 9.00 p.m., someone from Budleigh hospital telephoned my father (who was 85 at the time) and asked him when he would be moving his wife out of the hospital. My mother had been in the Budleigh hospital for just slightly more than 24 hours. No one there had made any attempt to make a diagnosis.

My father was startled and shocked by the suddenness and timing of the telephone call. He got the impression that the hospital was planning to send my mother home for him to look after by himself. My mother was doubly incontinent, required nursing on a ripple bed and had been diagnosed as demented. She had to be kept in a bed with cot sides so that she didn't fall onto the floor. On the odd occasion when she tried to feed herself, she ended up with food everywhere – with the result that both she and the bed had to be changed. My mother was so incapable of moving by herself that the nurses had a hoist and a bed lift fitted to the bed so that they could move my mother around and in and out of bed. It took two nurses to move her up the bed. She needed constant nursing attention.

My wife and I visited the hospital the next day, Thursday the 28th.

Within five minutes of my arriving at my mother's bedside, a nurse asked me to go to the sister's office where a rude and aggressive nurse demanded to know when my mother would be leaving the hospital. My mother had, by then, been in the hospital for no more than 48 hours. I found the questioning cruel, unfeeling and inhumane.

My father, who had been in a state of shock, now became depressed as a result of the hospital's attitude. Up until Monday the 25th April, my father had hoped that he would be able to have my mother back home or that, at the very least, he would be able to take her out of the hospital for trips in a wheelchair. He had been making plans to buy a motorised chair and a suitable vehicle so that he could do this.

When I spoke to the nurse at Budleigh Hospital on 28th April 2005, I was told that an assessment had been done and that my mother was considered fit to move out of the hospital and was now regarded as mentally alert. My mother had, according to Budleigh Hospital, been cured from her dementia within two days. She had received no new treatment. The nurse admitted that my mother needed nursing care but insisted that mentally there was nothing wrong with her. The hospital had, she told me, already applied for an enforcement order to have my mother removed from the hospital. I was shocked by their ruthlessness.

In reality, there had been no change whatsoever in my mother's condition. Several neurologists at Royal Devon and Exeter hospital had already agreed that my mother was suffering from severe dementia and though it turned out that they had missed the primary diagnosis, there wasn't much doubt that a diagnosis of dementia was accurate.

I complained about the fact that my father had been rung at home the evening before but the nurse didn't seem to think that there was anything wrong with that. She didn't apologise. I wanted to know just how ill you had to be to be in hospital these days. I felt overwhelmed with guilt. I had arranged for my mother to be moved to the Budleigh Hospital so that my father could visit more easily. And now they wanted to throw her out. But where could we take her? I went back to sit by my mother's bed. As I sat down my mother looked up and pointed to a stranger on the other side of the ward. 'Is that Vernon over there?' she enquired. We were living a nightmare. She didn't know who I was. She didn't recognise my wife. When I talked to her, she didn't even know that she was in hospital. Somewhere in the hospital a bell rang. 'There's someone at the door,' she said.

Someone at the Budleigh hospital threatened to send my mother home in an ambulance, even though they knew that my father could hardly look after himself let alone care for someone who needed intensive nursing care. My mother was, said one snotty, little bureaucrat, 'terminally but not finally terminally ill'. It was the first time I'd heard the phrase. My father, in his mid-80s, was devastated. 'What do I do if they send her home?' he asked. 'Don't answer the door,' I told him. 'Don't let them into the house. Call me.' I was telling my father to refuse to let the ambulance men bring my mother into the house. It was awful, just bloody awful. If the plan was to put us under pressure it was working very well. I'd never seen my father so distraught.

My mother's GP at the time agreed that we would not be able to find a local nursing home capable of looking after her. No one at the Budleigh hospital seemed to me to give a damn what happened to my mother as long as she wasn't their responsibility.

As far as I am aware, no one made the slightest attempt to make a diagnosis during the time my mother was in the Budleigh Hospital. Since they didn't want to nurse her and they didn't do any diagnostic tests, it was difficult to see the point of the hospital – apart from providing employment for the staff.

On the 11th May 2005, I had to attend a meeting at Budleigh hospital to discuss my mother's expulsion from the hospital. I was told that the hospital did not have enough beds and desperately needed to get rid of my mother. There were four people at the meeting: two members of the nursing staff, someone who looked like an administrator and Dr Taylor, my mother's GP at the time. The meeting was held in a completely empty ward. There were plenty of beds, all empty, and it seemed to me that this wasn't the first time the empty ward had been used for a meeting. If the hospital was short of anything it was patients, not beds.

The meeting lasted an hour and it was one of the most unpleasant hours of my life. It was not a meeting where the words 'compassion' and 'caring' figured large. I have been grilled by some of the country's toughest television and radio interviewers. I have given evidence in the House of Lords and the House of Commons but nothing prepared me for this. For a solid hour, the four of them battered at me to take my mother out of the hospital. They used every manipulative and emotional trick in the book. I quickly realised that no one there cared a damn about my mother or my father. They just wanted to get rid of a patient who seemed likely to be a long-term expense. This was business. I was still desperate to try to find a diagnosis. I was still trying to support my father. I was grieving for my mother who no longer even recognised me.

I was told that my mother would be better off in a nursing home and that the hospital didn't have any long-stay beds. I was told that they needed the bed for other patients (no one seemed to see the irony in the fact that the meeting was being held in a completely empty ward) and that my father would be better off if my mother was elsewhere. They didn't explain how this could be when there was no nursing home for miles that would be able to cope with her needs.

At the end of the meeting, I was told that they couldn't agree to my mother staying in the hospital and that she had to leave. I left the meeting and went back to my mother's bedside. She was still unable to move. She still didn't know who she was or where she was. She didn't know who I was. She was still faecally incontinent. She still had a catheter in her bladder to collect her urine. She still had to be fed. She still couldn't walk or even wash herself. But according to the hospital staff she was fine and mentally alert.

Ageism is the new racism: no respect, no consideration, no courtesy, no dignity, no caring.

For several weeks after that, my father didn't dare visit my mother at all. He was frightened that he would again be pressured by the staff to move my mother. He didn't know where he could take her. Overwhelmed with grief, he was now also tortured by guilt and anxiety.

Another mental assessment was done on my mother. It was a sick joke. The assessor asked my mother what I did for a living. My mother thought for a while. 'He's a teacher,' she said at last. She didn't know who I was, let alone what I did for a living. 'That's close enough,' answered the assessor putting a tick in another box. My mother was declared mentally competent.

Later that day, my father was sitting by my mother's side when the vicar called. My mother told him they were waiting for a train. The vicar thought it was a joke but my mother was serious. She kept asking my father why the train wasn't there and why there were dogs fighting in the ward. My mother didn't recognise my father (to whom she had been married for over 60 years) or know what he'd done for a living. She didn't even know who she was or where she was. She held her head a good deal and it was clear that she was having constant headaches. (No one at the hospital realised that these were caused by the increase in the amount of fluid surrounding her brain.)

On the 27th July, I attended another meeting in Budleigh Hospital. This time there were nine people there representing the hospital and the NHS. Dr Graham Taylor, my mother's GP was there, together with two nurses, a 'continuity care manager', an 'acting leading continuity nurse', a 'hospital care manager', a 'discharge facilitator', a representative of the administrators and a representative from Exmouth social services.

Someone began by saying that they all had my mother's best interests at heart. Someone else said they were delighted to report that my mother was much better and was improving. I asked them why, if this was the case, they weren't giving her any occupational therapy or physiotherapy. No one had an answer to this. I asked them how they had managed to produce this miracle without any treatment. I wanted to know how a woman who had been officially declared terminally ill and demented and in need of constant care, had suddenly become 'physically capable and mentally alert' after a few weeks in a small town hospital. No one had any answers.

In fact, of course, when the final diagnosis was made, it was quite clear that my mother could not possibly have shown any physical or mental improvement. She was suffering from idiopathic normal pressure hydrocephalus which was steadily getting worse. NHS staff who said that my mother had recovered and was no longer demented and could be discharged were lying because they wanted to throw her out of the hospital.

When I pointed out that my mother needed intensive nursing care, a continuity care manager claimed, to my utter astonishment, that catheters, hoists and ripple beds were not medical equipment. I asked him what would count as medical equipment. He said a ventilator would count as medical equipment. The phrase 'final stage terminal illness' was used. And again I heard the phrase 'terminally, terminally ill'. I asked how they knew that a patient was terminally, terminally ill, and was told that they could tell this through liver and kidney deterioration. I asked if they had done any tests to check on this, and it was generally agreed that they couldn't remember whether any such tests had been done.

I have no idea why nine people wasted a good chunk of a day on such a pointless meeting. I hate to think what it must have cost. It occurred to me as I sat there that if they were all sacked there would be plenty of money left for looking after patients. I told them that the bullying had won and that we would take my mother out of the hospital so that they could have yet another empty bed.

In the end my father couldn't bear it any longer. The staff at the Budleigh Hospital were making us feel so unwelcome, and harassing us so much, that we had no choice but to move my mother. As far as the NHS was concerned, it was all about money. They wanted to avoid the cost of looking after my mother – even though they had a moral and legal responsibility to do so. We found the Cranford Nursing Home, a private nursing home in Exmouth where for around £750 a week my mother had a private room which seemed crowded with three adults visiting. If a hotel had offered us the room, we would have walked out in disgust. Naturally, there were now no attempts to make a diagnosis.

My father sold his home and bought a small house near to the nursing home so that he could visit regularly.

Towards the end of her life we visited my mother in the nursing home and as soon as Antoinette entered the room, she turned to me and said that my mother had a swollen, bulging eye. (I believe that my wife had, by this time, more knowledge of idiopathic normal pressure hydrocephalus than the entire NHS medical staff in Devon.) The diagnosis was now beyond doubt. My mother had a bulging eye because of the pressure inside her skull. In idiopathic normal pressure hydrocephalus, the pressure within the skull remains normal because the expanding fluid volume compresses and destroys brain tissue. When the brain cannot be compressed any more, the fluid pressure must rise.

I contacted my mother's new GP and asked him to arrange for my mum to go back into Exeter hospital. Neither he nor any of the nursing home staff had noticed anything amiss.

In the Royal Devon and Exeter Hospital, the doctors at last confirmed the diagnosis of idiopathic normal pressure hydrocephalus. It was the diagnosis we'd offered them within days of my mother falling ill. Numerous consultants (including several neurologists), countless junior hospital doctors, one or two GPs and several dozen nurses all missed the diagnosis. If they'd acted within days or even weeks of her being admitted then they could have saved her life. We watched my mother die a terrible, slow death. She died because the doctors failed to make the diagnosis until it was too late.

The Royal Devon and Exeter hospital where my mother was treated so appallingly is a teaching hospital where medical students are turned into doctors.

Appendix Five

Homocysteine and Alzheimer's disease

Some authorities have linked the development of Alzheimer's disease to raised levels of homocysteine in the blood.

There still appears to be some mystery about this but I suspect that there shouldn't be.

The link is very straightforward.

The homocysteine levels in the blood rise when there is a shortage of vitamin B12. When vitamin B12 levels go down, homocysteine levels tend to go up. And vice versa.

Patients who are diagnosed as having Alzheimer's disease and who are then found to have raised homocysteine levels may have been misdiagnosed.

The chances are high that those patients don't have Alzheimer's at all but instead have an insufficiency of vitamin B12.

I suspect that when the shortage of vitamin B12 has been attended to, some or all of the symptoms of dementia will slowly disappear. And, miraculously, the Alzheimer's disease that was never there will have been cured.

Appendix Six

Dementia and high blood pressure

A widely reported study has claimed that a slightly increased blood pressure in middle life leads to an increased risk of developing dementia in later life.

As a result, doctors are now being encouraged to start treating more patients with drugs to lower their blood pressure. Doctors' surgeries will be busier than ever with doctors writing out prescriptions for millions of apparently healthy patients. Drug companies are no doubt worried about what they will do with all the extra money they will be making.

In fact, at this rate it surely won't be long before just about everyone over the age of 35 will be taking drugs to lower their blood pressure.

But does a slightly raised blood pressure really lead to more dementia?

I worry that this study may not show that at all.

What about all the possible variables?

So, for example, did the researchers weigh the patients involved throughout the period involved? Did they check their daily stress levels? Did they assess mental agility? Did they study smoking and drinking habits in detail? These may all be factors which are extremely relevant.

I understand that the patients involved in the study were all civil servants. That is a pretty closely selected group of individuals. Some civil servants tend not to have intellectually demanding or stimulating jobs. Could it be (as I suspect) that this might be a factor in the development of dementia?

And what effect will drug taking have on dementia? Is it really safe to take drugs to lower slightly raised blood pressure – especially if those drugs are to be taken for decades?

What about the risks of accidental hypotension – a common problem among those taking drugs for blood pressure. Could that be a serious problem for many of the millions who will now start taking drugs?

Personally, I fear that this is another piece of research best ignored.

(It rather reminds me of the research paper which showed that smokers did not develop dementia. The people who commented on that paper apparently didn't notice that many smokers never live beyond the age of 65 – and so never reach the age when dementia becomes commonest.)

The world's medical correspondents leapt on this research with great enthusiasm.

And I have no doubt that many apparently healthy individuals will now be taking medication for the rest of their lives.

Still, there will be one huge beneficiary from this research: the drug companies making pills to lower blood pressure.

This research will be worth billions to those pharmaceutical companies.

Appendix Seven

Paracetamol and Alzheimer's disease

In 1971, it was shown that phenacetin, a very popular but rather deadly painkiller, might cause Alzheimer's disease. This didn't matter very much because phenacetin had been banned because of the damage it did to the kidneys.

However, back in 1948, it had been shown that phenacetin is known to be converted into paracetamol in the body. The analgesic effect of phenacetin is a result of the paracetamol.

So, the big question, which, as far as I can find out no one has ever asked is: might paracetamol cause Alzheimer's disease?

The research is now forgotten and ignored. But it scared me because paracetamol is used daily by millions and is generally regarded as a safe drug.

And here's another scary thought.

Some decades ago, it was found that aspirin could cause an incredibly rare disease called Reye's Syndrome when it was given to children. And so it was recommended that children be given paracetamol instead of aspirin.

And the drug Calpol, which is widely used to ease mild pains in children, and also used by many parents as a sleeping aid, contains paracetamol.

Could it possibly be that all this explains the rising incidence of Alzheimer's disease? Could paracetamol be the cause of the fact that Alzheimer's is a common cause of dementia?

This worries the hell out of me.

And now it can worry the hell out of you because as far as I can find out no one is doing any research to find out.

Oh, and there's something else.

Guess which drug is now widely recommended for the treatment of patients with Alzheimer's disease.

Even though the preliminary evidence rather suggests that paracetamol could be the cause of Alzheimer's disease, the drug now widely prescribed for the treatment of the disease is – paracetamol.

There's a desperate need for some fairly simple research. It wouldn't take much work, time or money.

But researchers aren't interested. Most medical research is funded, directly or indirectly, by drug companies, and why would they want to do research which might dramatically reduce the number of patients needing expensive treatments?

To understand the world of medicine you have to understand how drug industry executives think.

Appendix Eight

Alzheimer's disease financial incentive

The incidence of dementia is about to rise exponentially now that British doctors are being paid a large bonus every time they diagnose Alzheimer's disease. I've told everyone I know to be on their toes when visiting their doctor. Too much hesitation and not enough blind certainty could well lead to an inconvenient diagnosis and a place of your own on the Involuntary Euthanasia Waiting List.

Medical journalists in the UK claim that this is the first time doctors have been paid to make a specific diagnosis but, as usual, they're wrong. British doctors have for years been given cash bonuses for diagnosing a wide range of disorders – including asthma, diabetes, heart disease and that artificial diagnostic confection known as 'COPD'.

It is, therefore, no surprise to discover that (officially at least) all these diseases are becoming commoner by the week.

Moreover, patients (and relatives) must take care to ensure that a diagnosis of Alzheimer's disease is not made when the real diagnosis should be the eminently treatable conditions of vitamin B12 deficiency or normal pressure hydrocephalus. Normal pressure hydrocephalus is dramatically underdiagnosed and is, I suspect, far commoner than most doctors believe. Doctors do not receive a fee for diagnosing normal pressure hydrocephalus or vitamin B12 – both of which commonly occur and both of which are curable but neither of which makes vast sums of money for drug companies.

Appendix Nine

Alzheimer's disease and death

Alzheimer's disease is officially regarded as a major killer. In the US it is said to be the fifth commonest killer of people over the age of 65. Doctors and journalists often describe patients as having died from Alzheimer's disease.

However, I have always struggled to understand why Alzheimer's disease should be a direct cause of death. Alzheimer's affects the brain, destroying connections and affecting a patient's ability to think, to remember, to eat, to walk and to do any of the things normally associated with life. But Alzheimer's disease does not stop a patient breathing and it does not stop the heart beating. By itself, Alzheimer's disease does not kill those who have it. You don't die of Alzheimer's disease any more than you die of confusion caused by a long-term tranquilliser overdose.

When patients are said to have died from Alzheimer's disease, they will have usually died of pneumonia or some other infection which has been deliberately left untreated. Or they may have had a stroke or some other circulatory incident which has resulted in death. In many cases, doctors and relatives will have chosen to allow the patient to die so that the suffering is ended.

There are, however, forms of dementia which can lead to death. So, for example, a patient who has genuinely died as a direct result of their dementia, without an infection or any other complication, may have died from idiopathic normal pressure hydrocephalus which was not diagnosed but which caused death by compressing, damaging and destroying many different parts of the brain. Alzheimer's disease does not do this. And vitamin B12 deficiency, which causes cerebral and spinal cord injury, can cause death if it has not been diagnosed (or treated properly).

I wonder how many of the patients whose deaths have been reported as being due to Alzheimer's disease were misdiagnosed and had actually been suffering from, and had died from, normal pressure hydrocephalus or vitamin B12 deficiency – both of which could have been cured.

Appendix Ten

When demented patients wander

Many patients with dementia have developed a tendency to wander. Relatives sometimes write and ask if I think it would be a good idea to have a patient fitted with an electronic tag so that they can be found quickly if they wander away from home. They worry, however, that it might be demeaning to do this. Safety is paramount and I think patients with dementia should be tagged – for everyone's benefit.

Indeed, I cannot see why all patients with dementia are not routinely offered an electronic tagging service.

It would be a better answer than the solution favoured in some British hospitals where patients with Alzheimer's are now handcuffed to their beds so that they do not require too much care and attention from the nurses.

Appendix Eleven

Recommendations

Don't accept a diagnosis of Alzheimer's disease until all other possible, treatable causes have been excluded.

In my opinion, the three specific disorders which must always be excluded before Alzheimer's disease is diagnosed are: prescription drug side effects; vitamin B12 deficiency and normal pressure hydrocephalus. Each of those disorders can be treated easily and quickly. I fear far too many patients are being mistakenly diagnosed as suffering from Alzheimer's disease – simply because this is the default diagnosis routinely adopted by family doctors.

And please remember that advice given by the medical establishment may well be wrong.

So, for example, in the UK, the advice given officially by the NHS is often inaccurate or misleading.

It is also vital to remember that the blood values used by laboratories are usually far too low.

The incidence of vitamin B12 deficiency is so common that even healthy individuals over 60 should have their B12 levels measured every three years or so.

Indeed, it would probably be wiser to give everyone over 60 vitamin B12 injections every three months. This would be much more useful than giving them all influenza shots.

It won't happen, of course.

There is far more profit to be made out of giving a vaccination than there is out of giving a vitamin B12 injection.

Dr Vernon Coleman MB ChB DSc FRSA, is the author of over 100 books – most of which are available on Amazon as paperbacks and as eBooks. For more information please see Dr Coleman's author page on Amazon or visit www.vernoncoleman.com where there are many free articles and no fees or advertisements.

If you found this book helpful Vernon Coleman would be very grateful if you would post a review online.

Printed in Great Britain
by Amazon